BEHAVIORAL SCIENCE
IN FAMILY PRACTICE

BEHAVIORAL SCIENCE IN FAMILY PRACTICE

Gerald M. Rosen, Ph.D.

Clinical Assistant Professor
Department of Family Medicine
School of Medicine
University of Washington
Seattle, Washington

John P. Geyman, M.D.

Professor and Chairman
Department of Family Medicine
School of Medicine
University of Washington
Seattle, Washington

Richard H. Layton, M.D.

Clinical Professor in Family Medicine
Director, Providence Family Medical Center
Seattle, Washington

APPLETON-CENTURY-CROFTS / New York

80 81 82 83 84 / 10 9 8 7 6 5 4 3 2 1

Prentice-Hall International, Inc., London
Prentice-Hall of Australia, Pty. Ltd., Sydney
Prentice-Hall of India Private Limited, New Delhi
Prentice-Hall of Japan, Inc., Tokyo
Prentice-Hall of Southeast Asia (Pte.) Ltd., Singapore
Whitehall Books Ltd., Wellington, New Zealand

Library of Congress Cataloging in Publication Data
Main entry under title:
Behavioral science in family practice.

  Bibliography: p.
  Includes index.
  1. Medicine and psychology.   2.   Family medicine—
Psychological aspects.   I.   Rosen, Gerald M., 1945–
II.   Geyman, John P., 1931–   III.   Layton, Richard H.,
1927–   [DNLM: 1.   Behavioral sciences.   2.   Family
practice.   WB110 B419.]
R726.5.B427   616'.001'9   79–23303
ISBN 0–8385–0638–0

PRINTED IN THE UNITED STATES OF AMERICA

BEHAVIORAL SCIENCE IN FAMILY PRACTICE

Gerald M. Rosen, Ph.D.

Clinical Assistant Professor
Department of Family Medicine
School of Medicine
University of Washington
Seattle, Washington

John P. Geyman, M.D.

Professor and Chairman
Department of Family Medicine
School of Medicine
University of Washington
Seattle, Washington

Richard H. Layton, M.D.

Clinical Professor in Family Medicine
Director, Providence Family Medical Center
Seattle, Washington

APPLETON-CENTURY-CROFTS / New York

80 81 82 83 84 / 10 9 8 7 6 5 4 3 2 1

Prentice-Hall International, Inc., London
Prentice-Hall of Australia, Pty. Ltd., Sydney
Prentice-Hall of India Private Limited, New Delhi
Prentice-Hall of Japan, Inc., Tokyo
Prentice-Hall of Southeast Asia (Pte.) Ltd., Singapore
Whitehall Books Ltd., Wellington, New Zealand

Library of Congress Cataloging in Publication Data
Main entry under title:
Behavioral science in family practice.

  Bibliography: p.
  Includes index.
  1. Medicine and psychology. 2. Family medicine—
Psychological aspects. I. Rosen, Gerald M., 1945–
II. Geyman, John P., 1931–   III. Layton, Richard H.,
1927–   [DNLM: 1. Behavioral sciences. 2. Family
practice. WB110 B419.]
R726.5.B427   616'.001'9   79–23303
ISBN 0–8385–0638–0

PRINTED IN THE UNITED STATES OF AMERICA

CONTRIBUTORS

Raymond C. Anderson, M.D.
Chairman and Associate Professor
Department of Family Medicine
Medical Center
University of California, Irvine
South Orange, California

Bill D. Burr, M.D.
Associate Professor
Department of Family Practice
School of Medicine
University of California, Davis
Davis, California

Hiram B. Curry, M.D.
Professor and Chairman
Department of Family Practice
College of Medicine
Medical University of South Carolina
Charleston, South Carolina

John P. Geyman, M.D.
Professor and Chairman
Department of Family Medicine
School of Medicine
University of Washington
Seattle, Washington

Nicholas T. Grace, M.D.
Assistant Clinical Professor
Division of Ambulatory & Community Medicine
School of Medicine
University of California at San Francisco
San Francisco, California

D. Daniel Hunt, M.D.
Assistant Professor
Department of Psychiatry and Behavioral Sciences
School of Medicine
University of Washington
Seattle, Washington

Arthur Kleinman, M.D.
Professor and Head, Psychiatric Consultation—Liaison Service
Department of Psychiatry and Behavioral Sciences
School of Medicine
University of Washington
Seattle, Washington

Thomas L. Leaman, M.D.
Professor and Chairman
Department of Family and Community Medicine
M.S. Hershey Medical Center
Hershey, Pennsylvania

John H. Leversee, M.D.
Associate Professor
Department of Family Medicine
School of Medicine
University of Washington
Seattle, Washington

George H. Lowrey, M.D.
Emeritus Professor of Pediatrics
School of Medicine
University of California, Davis
Davis, California

Ellen McGrath, Ph.D.
Assistant Professor of Psychiatry and Human Behavior
School of Medicine
University of California, Irvine
Orange, California

Edward Messner, M.D.
Assistant Clinical Professor
Department of Psychiatry
Harvard Medical School
Boston, Massachusetts

William R. Phillips, M.D., M.P.H.
Clinical Assistant Professor
Department of Family Medicine
School of Medicine
University of Washington
Seattle, Washington

Donald C. Ransom, Ph.D.
Associate Professor-in-Residence
Division of Ambulatory & Community Medicine
School of Medicine
University of California at San Francisco
San Francisco, California

Burton V. Reifler, M.D.
Assistant Professor
Department of Psychiatry and Behavioral Sciences
School of Medicine
University of Washington
Seattle, Washington

Jack Martin Reiter, M.D.
Clinical Assistant Professor
Department of Psychiatry and Behavioral Sciences
School of Medicine
University of Washington
Seattle, Washington

Gerald M. Rosen, Ph.D.
Clinical Assistant Professor
Department of Family Medicine
School of Medicine
University of Washington
Seattle, Washington

David D. Schmidt, M.D.
Associate Professor
School of Medicine
Case Western Reserve University
Cleveland, Ohio

John L. Shelton, Ph.D.
Diplomate in Clinical Psychology, Rehabilitation Medicine
School of Medicine
University of Washington
Seattle, Washington

Gabriel Smilkstein, M.D.
Associate Professor
Department of Family Medicine
School of Medicine
University of Washington
Seattle, Washington

Charles Kent Smith, M.D.
Associate Professor and Vice-Chairman
Department of Family Medicine
School of Medicine
University of Washington
Seattle, Washington

G. Gayle Stephens, M.D.
Professor and Chairman
Department of Family Practice
School of Medicine
University of Alabama in Birmingham
Birmingham, Alabama

Joe P. Tupin, M.D.
Professor and Chairman
Department of Psychiatry
School of Medicine
University of California, Davis
Davis, California

Reva K. Twersky, M.S.W.
Clinical Assistant Professor
Department of Family Medicine
School of Medicine
University of Washington
Seattle, Washington

Merrill N. Werblun, M.D.
Chairperson
Department of Family Practice
San Bernardino County Medical Center
San Bernardino, California

Richard M. Yarvis, M.D., M.P.H.
Clinical Associate Professor
Department of Psychiatry
School of Medicine
University of California, Davis
Davis, California

CONTENTS

Preface   xiii

Section I   **Defining Behavioral Science**

Chapter 1   The Behavioral Sciences in Family Medicine   3
G. Gayle Stephens

Chapter 2   A Model for Applying Behavioral Science to Family
Practice   15
Gabriel Smilkstein

Section II   **Individual and Family Development**

Chapter 3   Child Development   31
George H. Lowrey

Chapter 4   Adult Development   49
Thomas L. Leaman

Chapter 5   Family Development   67
John P. Geyman and Joe P. Tupin

Chapter 6   Clinical Applications of a Developmental
Framework   83
Charles Kent Smith, Jack Martin Reiter, and
Burton V. Reifler

Section III   **Approaches to Diagnosis**

Chapter 7   Psychosocial Issues in Assessment   95
Arthur Kleinman and Gabriel Smilkstein

Chapter 8   Basic Interviewing Skills   109
               Charles Kent Smith and John H. Leversee

Chapter 9   Interviewing the Difficult Patient   123
               David D. Schmidt and Edward Messner

Chapter 10   Assessment of Family Function   141
               Gabriel Smilkstein

Chapter 11   The Mental Status Examination   155
               Hiram B. Curry

Chapter 12   Self-Monitoring by Patients   171
               John L. Shelton and Gerald M. Rosen

Chapter 13   Psychological Testing   189
               William R. Phillips and Gerald M. Rosen

Section IV   **Approaches to Treatment**

Chapter 14   Applications of Counseling and Psychotherapy   203
               G. Gayle Stephens

Chapter 15   Crisis Intervention   217
               Richard M. Yarvis and Bill D. Burr

Chapter 16   Time-Limited Psychotherapy   231
               D. Daniel Hunt

Chapter 17   Family Therapy   247
               Donald C. Ransom and Nicholas T. Grace

Chapter 18   Use of Family Health Groups   265
               Ellen McGrath and Raymond C. Anderson

Chapter 19   Use of Community Resources   279
               Merrill N. Werblun and Reva K. Twersky

Index   291

PREFACE

In the ten years since Family Practice was recognized as the twentieth specialty in American medicine, remarkable progress has been made toward shaping the clinical, educational, and research dimensions of the specialty. One of the basic tenets of family practice has been the recognition of behavioral science as an essential part of family medicine. Family practice teaching programs, particularly at the graduate level, have stressed behavioral science and have included behavioral scientists on their staff. Despite this emphasis, the broadness of the field has led to debate concerning the content of behavioral science that is most relevant to the practice and teaching of family medicine. Varied definitions of behavioral science and different orientations have competed for attention and acceptance.

Although family medicine has wisely avoided premature closure in the definition of behavioral science, enough experience has been gained that some definition and structure is appropriate. *Behavioral Science in Family Practice* is an effort to present an organized framework for this diverse field. Section I of the book explores the background and historical roots of behavioral science in family practice, and provides a conceptual model for integrating behavioral science into family practice. Section II deals with individual and family development, since the heart of family medicine as a specialty is the ability to treat patients and their problems within a broader context. Sections III and IV follow naturally as sections on diagnosis and management.

The editors of this text represent varied backgrounds and viewpoints. Gerald M. Rosen, Ph.D., is a clinical psychologist in private practice who previously worked with Providence Family Medical Center, Seattle, as Behavior Science Coordinator. John P. Geyman, M.D., is Chairman of the Department of Family Medicine at the University of Washington and Editor of the *Journal of Family Practice*. He formerly practiced as a family physician in a small town. Richard H. Layton, M.D., who directs the residency training program at Providence Family Medical Center in Seattle, previously maintained a rural family practice for nineteen years. The editors feel that these varied orientations have broadened the book's view of behavioral science in family practice.

This book is intended for medical students interested in family medicine, family practice residents, and practicing family physicians. It should also be of interest to behavioral scientists and to many students and practitioners in the allied health fields. We hope that readers will see this book as an introduction to a variety of areas for further study. The book provides a framework and a springboard for active exploration of an emerging field.

GERALD M. ROSEN, PH.D.
JOHN P. GEYMAN, M.D.
RICHARD H. LAYTON, M.D.
SEATTLE, WASHINGTON

BEHAVIORAL SCIENCE
IN FAMILY PRACTICE

SECTION I

Defining Behavioral Science

CHAPTER 1

THE BEHAVIORAL SCIENCES IN FAMILY MEDICINE

G. GAYLE STEPHENS

Right at the beginning of the student's introduction to clinical medicine he should realize, and his teachers should emphasize, that illness is usually not an isolated event in a localized part of the body, but a change in a complex, integrated human being who lives and works in a particular social and family setting, and has a biological—psychological—social history.[1]

In addition to the traditional biological and clinical sciences, the program of preparation for family practice should have significant content in the behavioral sciences. The unique function of the family physician depends heavily upon adequate understanding of the behavioral sciences.[2]

It is clear from these two references taken from the two most important documents in the modern renaissance of family practice, that by the early 1960s our predecessors were recognizing the importance of a new element in the preparation of a physician for clinical practice— "behavioral science." Exactly how and why this new conviction came about has never, to my knowledge, been properly described.

Neither of the two reports specified what they meant by behavioral

3

science nor offered guidance about how to teach it. The Willard Report admitted:

> It is not clear at this time how best to incorporate the behavioral sciences in education for family practice . . . The proper role of behavioral science and the behavioral scientist in the medical center and in the practice of medicine remain to be defined.[3]

There was the suggestion that behavioral science had something to do with comprehensive care, holistic care, humanism in medicine, the physician's self-understanding, and possibly community medicine, but none of these terms were better defined academically than behavioral science itself.

These ideas are remarkable when it is noted that the committees making such recommendations represented organized medicine (The American Medical Association and The American Academy of General Practice) more than academic medicine. The Willard Committee was comprised almost entirely of practicing family physicians and it proposed stronger recommendations. There was one sociologist member of the Millis Commission but this can hardly account for the phenomenon under discussion.

Precisely what constitutes behavioral science and its relation to medical education and practice remains somewhat cloudy even now. There is no authoritative definition of the term and no section in medical libraries bearing that name; there is no section labeled family practice, but modern family practice educators have taken the recommendation seriously and have been trying to implement it for more than a decade. Since there is still no unanimity about the content of behavioral science, nor when and how it should be taught, it might be instructive to examine some of its roots in medicine. What follows represents the individual perspective of the author as an active participant in the family practice education movement over the past twelve years.

HISTORICAL ROOTS OF BEHAVIORAL SCIENCE IN FAMILY PRACTICE

Traditional General Practice

Unquestionably there is a strong tradition in general practice for elements of clinical medicine that would now be included in behavioral science. One important element is our collective memory that the general practitioner of the past "knew" patients and their families, and was adept in the art of medicine. There is a genre of writing in both clinical medicine and literature that focuses on the importance of the doctor-patient relationship and the methods of "psychotherapy" used by past practitioners of general medicine. The power of this literary tradition is still evident in the popularity of the television series, based on the parentalhealer figure of the physician, "Marcus Welby, M.D." In the well-known *Horse and Buggy Doctor* written in 1938, A. E. Hertzler, based on his practice from the turn of the century, devotes a chapter to his understanding of the medical and surgical problems of women.[4] Though not couched in the language of modern behavioral science, it is hard to find more profound insights into marriage and child rearing. He recognized the importance of the fear of pregnancy, the hatred that sometimes exists between men and women, and the grief that parents feel over the deaths or failures of their children. He knew the hazards these problems presented to surgeons failing to account for them when operating upon women who had pelvic pain.

While these doctors of the past did not survive the urbanization, bureaucratization, and institutionalization of medicine, their passing has been increasingly lamented, both by the public and the profession. There is the conviction that an essential element of medical practice was lost when it became more specialized in the interests of science, and patients were forced to turn to a number of doctors for care, none of whom "knew" them as did the general practitioner. Excessive fragmentation and impersonality of care are persistent criticisms of modern medicine. When physicians and others became politically and educationally active in the 1960s on behalf of a restoration of the generalist role in medicine, they wanted to recover the lost wholeness and humanism. Behavioral science was appropriated as an academically legitimate vehicle by which this could be accomplished. Although they had no clear notion of how behavioral science should be incorporated into medical education, they were clear about what they hoped it could do.

Organizational Activities

The American Academy of General Practice* (American Academy of Family Physicians), established a Mental Health Committee ". . . to work with the American Psychiatric Association in developing programs of con-

---

* The author is grateful for permission to review the unpublished 1957–1967 annual reports of the Mental Health Committee to the Board of Directors of the American Academy of General Practice (AAFP after 1969). Material in this section was taken from these reports.

tinuing education in psychiatric techniques for general practitioners and maintain a liaison with other national associations in the field of mental health.[5]" The professional society of general practitioners recognized and moved to support a national policy on mental health that began in the 1950s and was in full swing in the 1960s. The establishment of the National Institute of Mental Health (NIMH), the funding of psychiatric graduate training through grants, and ultimately the creation of community mental health centers reflected that policy.

Initially the liaison efforts focused on teaching appropriate techniques of psychological treatment to general practitioners. The "workshop," then a novelty, was the method used. Psychiatrists served as leaders of meetings attended mainly by general practitioners. This method met with enthusiasm and success on a local, state, and regional basis. Funds were provided for these meetings by NIMH beginning in 1962 and continued until 1975. By 1969, the annual report of the Mental Health Committee stated: "There are so many courses being given each year that it is impossible to keep track of them all."

In 1965 the Mental Health Committee recognized the existence of the new Committee on Requirements for Certification (CORC) established by the Academy to promote the creation of a certifying examination for general practitioners. This was the forerunner of the American Board of Family Practice, established in 1969. The "core content" examination had an important section on psychiatry and mental health.

The first mention of the term "behavioral science" appeared in the Committee's 1970 annual report. By that time the change of name from general to family practice had occurred and there were 46 approved residencies in the new discipline. The AAFP Commission on Education had by then preempted the educational functions for mental health, both at the graduate and postgraduate levels, and the Committee on Mental Health began to play a secondary role. However, the NIMH grant was renewed for three years, 1973–1975, with the overall goals for future workshops to promote an understanding of (1) mental health problems in family practice; (2) behavioral sciences in family practice; (3) psychological aspects of medical diseases; and (4) basic psychiatric education for family physicians.

In view of the occupational stresses in that vocation, after 1975 the Mental Health Committee turned its attention to the mental health of family physicians. The "impaired physician" became the focus of workshops; new policies and procedures were developed to assist and rehabilitate impaired physicians instead of merely punishing them; and the teaching of patient treatment techniques was left to the educators in the new family practice residencies. This sketchy review of a great deal of activity indicates the degree to which the modern family practice movement was tied to an emerging national consciousness of mental health problems and to responsible institutions and organizations. Psychiatry and, later, behavioral sciences were seen as relevant to these issues.

Influence of Educational Psychology

A parallel movement to academic family medicine was the incorporation of educational psychology into medical education. Medical schools in the United States, perhaps to a greater extent than other professional schools, have been receptive to the theory and practice of professional educators. This occurred as medical teaching moved beyond the preceptoral model—partly in response to the need to teach increased numbers of medical students and partly in the interest of better educational quality control. Educational psychology is another root of academic behavioral science in modern medicine. Learning theory and the concept of developmental stages and tasks are readily identifiable elements of this discipline, which apply to patient care and not only to teaching and learning in school.

Family medicine, perhaps because of its newness in the academic setting, has been influenced greatly by educational psychology and all its residencies are required to have written objectives and methods of evaluation as criteria for accreditation. Much credit for beginning this interdisciplinary activity is due to Dr. Lynn Carmichael, Miami, Florida, who for several years around 1970 sponsored an annual winter meeting of the new family physician teachers, where professional educators from Michigan State University introduced them to educational psychology and methodology. These meetings were antecedents to the organization of the Society of Teachers of Family Medicine, an interdisciplinary body including not only physicians but academic social scientists, educators, psychologists, administrators, and medical social workers. It would be hard to overestimate the importance of this organization in the development and dissemination of behavioral science knowledge in family medicine.

British General Practice

A less formal but no less important influence on American general practice came from British general practice, which had never suffered the attrition in numbers or in academic development affecting their American counterparts. Notable among the British contributions was the work of Dr. Michael Balint, a psychoanalyst who developed a new form of the continuous case seminar for teaching about the doctor-patient relationship and focal psychotherapy to general practitioners. Balint's influence in the United States was mediated largely through the Department of Psychiatry at the University of Cincinnati School of Medicine, to which he came biannually for a number of years to hold short-term training seminars. Balint's book, *The Doctor, His Patient and the Illness*, is considered by some to be the definitive work on the doctor-patient relationship.[6] It has been widely used in family medicine education.

Clinical Pastoral Education

Clinical pastoral education via hospital chaplains has contributed another element of behavioral science to family medicine and to the rest of medicine. There are a number of similarities between the roles of pastor and family physician. Both are oriented towards the family and both participate in the rituals and crises of people's lives—birth, marriage, sickness, and death. They are essentially supportive and depend for their effectiveness upon the quality of personal relationships. Since many of the community hospitals that sponsored family practice residencies also employed chaplains, it was natural that some of them should have cooperated educationally as well as in patient care.

A major contribution from clinical pastoral education to family practice is a method of supervision of trainees known as the "verbatim." In this method the trainee presents to a supervisor a verbatim account, either written or tape recorded, of a clinical encounter with a patient. Modifications of this type of intensive, individual, and group supervision around professional conduct and communications have become almost universal in family medicine education. The focus is on the clinical work of the trainee rather than his individual mental health. It is a powerful tool in humanizing medical care and exposing professional insensitivity. The reader should not conclude that pastoral educators are alone in using these supervisory techniques; psychiatrists and psychologists use similar methods. However, chaplains were among the first to bring these methods to the attention of several of the pioneer family physician educators.

Another important contribution from clinical pastoral education is the management of grief and death. Hospital chaplains have developed a creditable body of literature about death and dying that has broad implications for all physicians.

Administrative Needs

Administrative science is another link to behavioral science in family medicine. It is widely recognized that problems in the organization and delivery of medical care may be more inimical to the patients' best interests than failures in communication by individual physicians. Both patients and physicians are constrained by the systems in which they come together. Practice management, therefore, has become an essential element of the family medicine curriculum; a new generation of professionally educated managers and administrators has joined the family practice team, bringing with them the principles and methods of organizational structure, industrial psychology, personnel management, and related subjects. This represents another application from the academic social sciences to behavioral science in medical practice.

These historical phenomena have been instrumental in bringing modern concepts of behavioral science to family practice. Given such diverse roots it is not surprising that a universal understanding of behavioral science has not emerged. What is remarkable is that so many influences converged in the late 1960s and early 1970s to give impetus to behavioral science in the new discipline of family medicine. It is now appropriate to examine the content of the major contributions.

THE INTELLECTUAL ROOTS OF BEHAVIORAL SCIENCE

The intellectual roots of contemporary behavioral science are diverse but four themes can be traced that have provided the research base from which all of the applied disciplines have drawn freely. These are (1) medical psychology and psychoanalysis; (2) the academic social sciences (anthropology, sociology, social psychology and psychology) (3) educational psychology and (4) metaphysics and religion. This classification is somewhat arbitrary, but useful, in making sense out of a rapidly expanding body of knowledge. A brief description of the contributions from each model will show that what we now call behavioral science is a generic term referring to elements from all four models. This description will hopefully reassure the reader that the subject is neither incomprehensible nor purely subjective, and that critical judgment is needed to identify the components that are most clinically applicable.

Medical Psychology and Psychoanalysis

Although psychoanalysis has never been popular within general medicine as a complete system for understanding patient behavior or as a method of treatment, it has made important contributions to medical psychology and practice. Some of its contributions have become so widely accepted that it is easy to overlook their origin. Psychoanalytic ideas are firmly entrenched in our culture and have been better expressed in novels and plays than in medicine. Concepts such as instinct, stages of development, intrapsychic conflict, defense mechanisms, repression, guilt, unconscious motivation, "family romances," fantasies, and complexes are part of our culture. Psychoanalysis also deals better than other models with the irrational or absurd dimensions of human behavior. It is unfortunate that the field became so identified with the language of mythology, interpretation of dreams and lengthy complex methods of treatment that the average physician rejected it as irrelevant or impossible to apply in medical practice.

Psychoanalysis provides a theoretical base for understanding the doctor-patient relationship and for establishing continuity of care. It recognizes the symbolic nature of that relationship through its concepts of transference and countertransference; and it deals with issues of autonomy, dependence, fear, anger, and eroticism within professional relationships. These ideas are essential to the maintenance of appropriate long-term supportive relationships, compliance, handling of elective medical and surgical procedures, scheduling, and fee payment. All of these are important to the work of family physicians, who are particularly exposed to the difficulty of time and uncertainty in medical practice, and deal more with personal services than technical procedures. The family physician who has a clear, cognitive appreciation for psychoanalysis has a firm foundation for clinical work, self-understanding, practice management, and utilization of other models of behavioral science.

Psychoanalytic interest in the history of the individual and origins of neuroses and psychoses in infantile experience has been incorporated into the study of constitutional and genetic factors in the epidemiology of mental illnesses, especially family studies of schizophrenia. Psychoanalytic interest in instinct and the unconscious has been superceded by the development of ego psychology and the recognition of the importance of conscious and interpersonal factors. The interest in the stages of infantile sexuality has been extended to include developmental stages throughout an individual's lifetime. The emphasis on the Oedipus stage of parent-child relationships includes the entire range of family life experiences. These statements do not constitute an intellectual history of psychoanalysis; they are meant to illustrate the broad scope of medical psychology, its debt to psychoanalysis, and the relevance of all these factors in any proper comprehension of behavioral science.

The Academic Social Sciences

The academic social sciences, including at least anthropology, sociology, social psychology, and clinical psychology, have been major contributors to modern behavioral science. Contributions have ranged from basic research to the generation of new professional disciplines such as medical social work, marriage counseling, family therapy, and group therapy. Medical psychology tended to focus on the individual and usually assumed a disease model of individual pathology, the academic social sciences take the intimate social relationships of the individual as their object of study and focus on individual interactions and communications within a group. They are more concerned with adaptation than pathology and, on the whole, take into account a larger number of variables than medical psychology.

Fundamental to all the social sciences is the work of George Herbert Mead,[7] who in the first thirty years of this century began to teach about the social nature of the self. Mead took the self as his object of study and showed that it is a uniquely human characteristic developing only within the context of social relationships. Mead's work opened new fields of study that are still being actively researched. Important among these is the nature of the two-person relationship or dyad and occurring interactions. In the dyad there are three entities, the two individuals and the relationship between them, a primary example in social theory of how the whole is more than the sum of its parts.

A second major contributor to social theory was George Homans[8] who studied the characteristics of small groups—families, street gangs, and workers in a plant—and laid the foundations for small group dynamics. Students of Mead and Homans extended their studies and added contributions from animal psychology (ethology), mathematics (game theory), anthropology, engineering (systems theory), linguistics, and semantics. From these have come new understandings of human behavior, having broad applications in medicine.

A Harvard biochemist, L. J. Henderson,[9] of the Henderson-Hasselbach equation, was among the first to teach that the practice of medicine could be understood as applied sociology. A follower of the Italian sociologist Pareto, Henderson taught medical students a course about this concept in the 1930s. Since then, a growing number of scholars have investigated: illness as a social role; psychotherapy; the influence of poverty, class and ethnic variables on medical epidemiology; marriage and child rearing; and death. The modern mental health movement is largely derived from these studies, though it also has roots in medical psychology. Family therapy is another derivative, combining role theory, communications theory, and systems theory. Transactional analysis is a combination of psychoanalysis with game theory. Other psychotherapies also represent the social scientists' contributions to health problems.

There are obvious overlaps and a common research base between educational psychology and academic social sciences. There are two aspects of educational psychology deserving special mention in a chapter devoted to the origin of behavioral science. The word "behavior" in its psychological sense is largely derived from experimental psychology and its descendent, learning theory. If medical psychology focused on the individual, and the social sciences focused on the self, experimental psychology from the time of Watson focused on behavior. The towering contemporary figure of B. F. Skinner has influenced generations of academic psychologists and his work is increasingly applied in medical care settings. From his laboratory work with animals, Skinner developed a powerful system of explanations and methods for modifying, changing or controlling animal behavior, including that of humans. The clinical application of learning theory utilizes a contingency system of rewards or punishments to affect targeted behaviors. It is widely utilized in health settings to deal with habits, addictions, obesity, and a variety of other symptoms. In biofeedback, it is used to control certain autonomic conditions such as hypertension, vascular headaches, and gastrointestinal symptoms.

Developmental Psychology

It is theoretically related to experimental psychology and behaviorism, but focuses more on the education of children. Along with psychoanalysis, developmental psychology has emphasized the concept of developmental stages and tasks. However, it has done this from an educational rather than a psychosexual perspective. It has contributed significantly to the management of learning disorders and mental retardation on the one hand, and to special education and residential schools on the other. Childhood autism has been of special interest. Well-known theorists and practitioners include Jean Piaget, Erik Erikson, Robert Havighurst and Bruno Bettelheim. Contributions to medical education from educational psychology have already been mentioned.

Humanistic Psychology and Religion

The fourth theme in modern behavioral science consists of a variety of strange theoretical bedfellows held together by a common interest in the person as distinct from previously identified interests in the individual, the self, and behavior. Person entails a different level of abstraction, and is uniquely concerned with the meaning of human experience; hence the frequent use of the term *existential* to apply to the dimension of meaning. The person is less concerned with freedom from individual pathology adaptation or conditioned responses than with fulfillment and the relief from alienation.

Sometimes referred to as "third force psychology," psychology of the person is clearly distinguishable from experimental or developmental psychology, and has been practiced and taught mainly outside of academic departments of psychology. We are indebted to Abraham Maslow for such concepts as "hierarchy of personal needs," "peak experiences," and "self actualization," while Gestalt psychology was popularized by Fritz Perls. Carl Rogers, in his later years, Rollo May, and Erich Fromm should also be mentioned as psychologists who bridged the gap from psychoanalysis and academic psychology to psychology of the person. More recently practitioners have turned to eastern religions for techniques of meditation and yoga.

There is clearly a religious streak in the psychology of the person, much of which can be traced to the nineteenth-century Danish philosopher, Soren Kierkegaard. Some of the European psychiatrists who survived Nazi concentration camps in the late 1930s or early 1940s developed methods of psychotherapy that seem more akin to salvation than cure. Viktor Frankl belongs to this genre; and the Swiss psychiatrist, Paul Tournier, is overtly religious in his therapy.

Psychology of the person certainly has had a perceptible influence on medical educators and practitioners, though its qualifications as science may be more open to skepticism than the three other themes previously discussed.

SUMMARY

What has been attempted in this chapter is the identification of a number of components and antecedents of the generic term, behavioral science; and a description of how these components were introduced to the developing new medical discipline, family medicine. The author takes no credit for originality and makes no claim for completeness in this account. It will be enough if the reader comes to appreciate the diversity of the contributions and contributors to a contemporary understanding of human behavior and recognizes the unfinished nature of the task. No current theory or method is adequate to deal with all clinical problems that affect our patients and ourselves.

The physician must select from this smorgasbord of "sciences" and "psychologies" those elements that make the most sense and are most useful clinically. Medical psychology surely is the basic behavioral science for physicians but it too is incomplete. The physician needs theories that go beyond medical preoccupation with diseases of individuals. Many of the behaviors that have impact upon health are not best conceived as diseases, but as problems of living. People live in groups, especially in families or family-like groups; and the locus of ill health is as frequently between or among intimates as within the individual. Many professionals other than physicians know a great deal about the characteristics of human togetherness, and how this influences the development of an individual. We would do well to learn from them.

REFERENCES

1. Millis J (chmn): *The Graduate Education of Physicians: The Report of the Citizens Commission on Graduate Medical Education.* Chicago: AMA, 1966
2. Willard WR (chmn): *Meeting the Challenge of Family Practice: The Report of the Ad Hoc Committee on Education for Family Practice.* Chicago: AMA, 1966
3. Willard: *Op. Cit.*
4. Hertzler AE: *The Horse and Buggy Doctor.* Lincoln: University of Nebraska Press, 1938
5. "Annual Reports of Mental Health Committee to Board of Directors, American Academy of General Practice" (after 1969, American Academy of Family Physicians), unpublished
6. Balint M: *The Doctor, His Patient and the Illness.* New York: International University Press, 1957
7. Strauss A (ed): *George Herbert Mead on Social Psychology.* Chicago: The University of Chicago Press, 1956, rev. 1964
8. Homans G: *The Human Group.* New York: Harcourt, Brace & Co., 1950
9. Barber B (ed): *L. J. Henderson on the Social System.* Chicago: University of Chicago Press, 1970

CHAPTER 2

A MODEL FOR APPLYING BEHAVIORAL SCIENCE TO FAMILY PRACTICE

GABRIEL SMILKSTEIN

INTRODUCTION

Balint's[1] book on the interaction between British general practitioners and their patients reveals the full range of the doctor-patient relationship. The spectrum reaches from those physicians who are "apostolic" in their management of patient problems (i.e., physicians who attempt to convert patients to their point of view), to those who attempt an in-depth understanding of their own feelings as well as those of their patients.

The material for Balint's book was drawn from seminars the author held with a group of general practitioners. The seminar discussions demonstrated how a host of transference and countertransference phenomena influenced the physician's approach to patient care. The seminar participants revealed that responses such as anger, fear, and sexual attraction overtly and covertly influenced the doctor-patient relationship. This information was not new to patient interviewers, but Balint used the knowledge to highlight the need for physicians to take stock of their emotional responses while interacting with patients.

Medical behavioral science is the study of the doctor-patient relationship as it pertains to (1) the role of the physician as the facilitator of health care and (2) the patient faced with a physical and/or psycho-social health problem who seeks assistance. The doctor-patient relationship is a complex of biomedical and psychosocial interactions that is significantly influenced by a host of variables. These variables include family and community, as well as social, cultural, economic, educational, and medical factors.

In general, the physician who holds to the biomedical model of health care avoids the complexity of psychosocial influences on the doctor-patient relationship. The biomedical model narrows the physician's charge to identifying and treating a disease process. It limits the patient's response to revealing those data that are pertinent to the identification and assessment of the disease process. Although the biomedical model is appealing because of its clear lines of responsibility, there is a growing literature that suggests it is inadequate for the scientific tasks and social responsibilities of medicine.[2, 3, 4]

A comprehensive approach to medicine is needed that views the patient within the milieu of family and community and gives credence to sociocultural influences.[5] The role of family medicine in developing such an approach is well stated by Mauksch.[2]

> The emergence of Family Medicine is symptomatic of a complex sense of discomfort within the health profession and by the public at large regarding the depersonalization and episodal discontinuity associated with the scientific advances of clinical medicine. . . . Family Medicine is associated with an almost cyclical rediscovery of the human, social and cultural aspects of health and illness and also with the growing concern about the gap between medical capabilities and the ultimate effectiveness of medical intervention.

If family medicine is to assume the mantle of integrator of the behavioral sciences into health care, a conceptual and empirical model is needed upon which teachers and practitioners can focus. The purpose of the present chapter is to present such a model.

A CONCEPTUAL AND EMPIRICAL MODEL OF BEHAVIORAL SCIENCE

The aid of a family physician is usually sought when a crisis renders a patient dysfunctional. Most crises require the family physician to intervene as a resource person for the management of disease and injury problems. In these cases, a measure of sensitivity is needed by the physician to recognize and respond to the patient's health beliefs[6] and illness behavior,[7] but an in-depth behavioral study is usually not required.

There are times, however, when the stress of psychosocial life events induces a loss of equilibrium or a state of dysfunction in a member of a family. The physician wishing to respond to the needs of such a patient requires an understanding of such medical behavioral science components as: (1) family function; (2) the impact of family crisis; (3) coping mechanisms; and (4) resource identification in crises. The conceptual model for considering these components in family practice is depicted in Figure 2-1.

The following outline highlights the basic features of the model:

I. Family in health: family members cope by using an active and available system of intra- and extrafamilial resources.
   A. Family life style is characterized by adaptive mechanisms chosen by the family and based on sociocultural heritage and milieu.[9, 10]
   B. Coping band of family members represents the range of functional variation which the family can manage while utilizing its own resources. The width of the coping band depends on the level of family function (i.e., the higher the level of function, the wider the band).
II. Family in trouble: members require help (unable to cope), i.e., stressful life events occur that require resources beyond those available to the family.
   A. A crisis exists when a family is unable to adapt within its coping band.
   B. The depth of dsyfunction that follows a crisis depends on the significance of the crisis.
   C. The significance of a crisis, or family value orientation[11] towards crisis, is based on: (1) previous experience with similiar crises; (2) sociocultural attitudes toward the crisis[7-10]; (3) role changes in family caused by the crisis; and (4) intra- and extrafamilial resources available to the family at the time of the crisis.[12]
III. The family members seek help: e.g., the family physician is activated as a resource.
   A. Communication is established between family members and family physician.
   B. Data base is obtained by the family physician who: (1) identifies crisis; (2) establishes significance of crisis; (3) determines level of family function; and (4) assesses resources available to family.
   C. Angle of recovery[13] reflects the family physician's ability to facilitate a program that will allow the family members to: (1) identify problems; (2) improve communication within and between the family and community; and (3) utilize available resources for problem-solving.

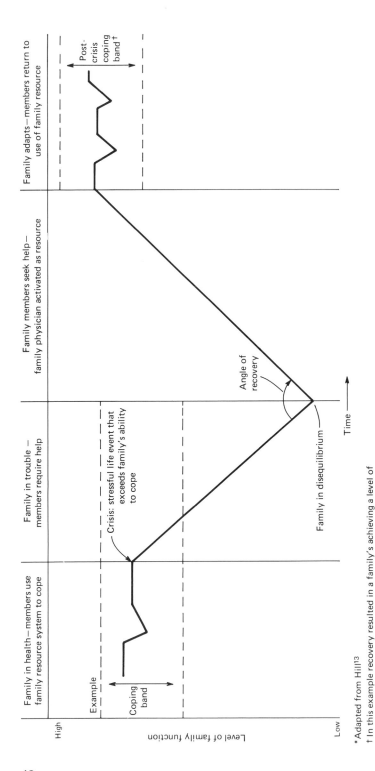

FIGURE 2-1. A conceptual model for applying the behavioral sciences to problems in family medicine.

*Adapted from Hill[13]

† In this example recovery resulted in a family's achieving a level of function higher than the pre-crisis level. According to the impact of crisis and resources available to a family many levels of recovery or non-recovery are possible.

18

TABLE 2-1.   Areas of Study for Psychosocial Problems in Family Medicine

Conceptual Model	Areas of Study
Family in health	Family function Family life cycle Family and child development Coping band
Family in trouble	Crisis/stressful life events Significance of crisis Family equilibrium Role change
Family members seek help	Communication concepts/problems Psychosocial and cultural explanatory models Illness problems/behavior Health belief models Identification of extrafamilial resources Family resources Therapeutic modalities: individual, group, and family therapy; family life; education
Family adapts, members return to use of personal resources	Family rituals Promoting family health

IV. Family members return to use of normal intra- and extrafamilial social support resources.
   A. A new level of family function is established.
   B. Preventive measures are taken to promote family health and to insure future integrity of the family (e.g., parenting education).

Table 2-1 demonstrates the areas of study relating to specific components of the conceptual model.

STRESSFUL LIFE EVENTS

In general, families that are highly functional with good lines of communication and available resources can manage stress through a wide range of intensity. On the contrary, dysfunctional families, characterized by poor communication and resources, have a limited capacity to cope. As a consequence, these families are more likely to use the health care system as a resource for coping with illness problems.[12-15]

Much has been written by the social scientists about the significance of stressful life events on the health status of individuals and their families,[16, 17] and the adaptive or coping mechanisms that may be employed.[18] An exciting area for future family medicine research is the study of families that demonstrate consistent patterns of illness without a biomedical explanation. Miller and Huygen[19, 20] have identified such cohorts of families, but a clear causal relationship between family dysfunction and recurrent illness has not yet been established.

PSYCHOSOCIAL CRISIS

Crisis is defined in this chapter as stressful life events, past and present, that produce psychosocial disequilibrium or dysfunction in an individual, in the relationship among family members, or in the relationship between family and community. Crises may be divided categorically into normative and nonnormative. Normative crises are life events that are part of the planned, expected, or normal processes of family life. Nonnormative crises are due to unexpected or adverse life experiences; consequently, they tend to have greater impact on family function than do normative crises.

External nonnormative crises (i.e., man-made and natural disasters such as wars and earthquakes) cause crises that usually result in transient family dysfunction. Families seem to respond to external crises with a rapid pooling of resources enabling members to function and survive under difficult circumstances. The level of family function achieved after recovery from nonnormative external crises is often higher than the precrisis level. This high level of family function, however, may deteriorate once the threat to survival is eliminated. Evidently, a less stressful life situation requires less resource sharing and lower levels of family member interaction.

Nonnormative internal crises such as marital infidelity, divorce, alcoholism, and criminal activity usually disrupt family function more than external crises. These crises are usually associated with extended periods of family dysfunction during which members have difficulty communicating and identifying resources necessary to resolve the crisis. Recovery, if it occurs, is usually delayed and often fails to reach the precrisis level of family function.

The family physician who wishes to establish a foundation for dealing with crises in clinical practice will find an excellent starting point in Hill's[13] generic explanation of crises. Table 2-2 divides life crises into normative and nonnormative components and lists crises under four generic categories:

TABLE 2-2.   Crises in Family Life

Normative	Nonnormative
Addition	
Adoption Assimilation of relative or friend into a household Birth Marriage	Assimilation of stepfather, stepmother, and/or stepsiblings into a family Unplanned pregnancy
Abandonment	
Elderly family member or friend dies Loss of function of family member due to minor illness Member(s) of peer group move away or find new friends Planned departure of family member (child leaves for camp, job, school; extended trip)	Child banished from family or ran away Family member or friend engaged in life-threatening activity (e.g., war) Family member or friend hospitalized or institutionalized Man and woman involved in desertion, divorce, or separation Sudden or violent death of family member or friend
Demoralization	
Rebellion against social norms and/or rules of family or community	Alcoholism or drug abuse Delinquency Infidelity or sexual aberration Jail sentence School expulsion
Status Change	
Admission to or departure from club, fraternity, political office, sorority Move to another community or school New stage of life (teenager, parent, middle-age, senior citizen) Raise in salary and/or position within current job Role change (job change, mother goes to work, single to married, school level change) Success or failure in gaining goals (academic degree, business contract, prize, or sports team position)	Acquisition or elimination of a physical or emotional handicap Change in living environment to or from different social strata (car, neighborhood, house) Loss of freedom (jail sentence, refugee status) Loss of income School expulsion Sudden fame or wealth

Source: Smilkstein G: "The Family in Crisis." In Taylor R (ed): *Family Medicine—Principles and Practices.* New York: Springer Verlag 1978, p. 235.

1. Addition is a crisis initiated by the short- or long-term addition of one or more members to the family structure.
2. Abandonment is associated with the threat of loss or the actual departure of a family member. Abandonment may also relate to the threat or actual loss of function that results in a significant role change for a family member.
3. Demoralization is a crisis that occurs when a family member initiates a change in the previously ordained family moral code.
4. Status change is a crisis in which a family member gains or loses wealth, power, or position.

Identifying and labeling a psychosocial crisis is of value to the physician involved in the work-up of a family in trouble. Of greater consequence, however, is an evaluation of the significance of a crisis to the family. Kluckholn[11] equates the significance of a crisis with the family's "value orientation." Sometimes a single crisis may have a high enough value orientation to bring a family member to the physician for help. More frequently, the accumulative stress of several crises will cause the dysfunction that requires professional assistance.

To ascertain the significance of a crisis, or the family member's value orientation toward a crisis, the physician must ask questions that reveal how the crisis has affected family function (see Chapter 10). Other data of value are past experiences with a similar crisis, role changes induced by the crisis, adaptive or coping mechanisms employed, and resources available to the family for the resolution of the crisis.

For example, a family whose only wage earner and family leader experiences a myocardial infarct would be maximally stressed if: (1) the family had a history of members who died from heart disease; (2) the members were already burdened with a number of other unresolved family crises; and (3) the family was new to the community and resource poor (e.g., new members of the community without a social support group).

Case Illustration

Tracing the assessment and management of a family through the behavioral science conceptual model can clarify the role of the family physician when managing a psychosocial crisis.

The identified patient, Cynthia, is a 14-year-old junior high school student who was referred to a University Family Medical Center following an attempted suicide. The patient was physically well-developed for her years and stated that she took the aspirin overdose because her parents would not allow her to date her 20-year-old boyfriend. She claimed loneliness and frustration as a result of her parents' restrictiveness. Cynthia stated that she was unable to talk to her mother about sex or anything else because there was no trust between them.

Cynthia's parents came to the Family Medical Center to discuss their daughter's problem. Cynthia's father, age 51, was an executive who spent long hours at work but apparently had a good relationship with his wife of 17 years. He delegated much of the responsibility for Cynthia's care to his wife. He claimed that his few attempts to discipline Cynthia had led to disagreeable confrontations.

Cynthia's mother, age 56, played the role of housewife and mother. She participated in art activities as her avocation. She had two daughters, ages 27 and 32, from a previous marriage who were married and out of the home. Cynthia's mother expressed a great fear for Cynthia's safety, explaining that a woman had been attacked in a park near their home. She had required that Cynthia be at home before dark, or call in if late. Cynthia was "grounded" whenever she failed to meet house rules.

Cynthia's parents felt that they were giving her "everything" and they could not understand their daughter's attitude of rebellion. A family conference was scheduled to initiate a more complete assessment of family function.

Family Function Data Base

1. Basic activities (work, study, sleeping and eating). The parents were apparently able to function satisfactorily—the father at his executive position and the mother in her art classes. Cynthia had been an elementary school honor student, but was currently failing most of her classes. Cynthia's mother claimed some sleep problems.
2. Communication. Cynthia's mother claimed that communication with her husband was good, depending upon his mood. Cynthia had major communication problems with her parents; she argued with her father and frequently lied to her mother. Cynthia's mother stated that Cynthia was sometimes difficult to reach.
3. Resources. This family had a network of social support persons, but many of the relationships seemed superficial. Family problems were not shared with individuals outside the family. Economic, education, and medical resources were judged as very satisfactory.
4. Family APGAR. The Family APGAR questionnaire is discussed more fully in Chapter 10. The questionnaire revealed that the husband-wife subsystem was functioning well, but the parent-child subsystem was highly dysfunctional. This was reflected in the following comments:

CYNTHIA:
I don't get along with Dad. My family does not get along and never will for that matter—maybe we could if we tried.

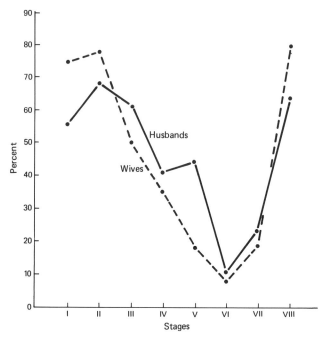

FIGURE 2-2.   Percentage of individuals in each stage of the family life cycle reporting their present stage of the family life is very satisfying. (Stage I, beginning families; Stage II, child-bearing families; Stage III, families with prseschool children; Stage IV, families with school-age children; Stage V, families with teenagers; Stage VI, families as launching center; Stage VII, families in the middle years; Stage VIII, aging families.) Source: Rollins BC and Feldman H: Marital satisfaction over the family cycle. J Mar Fam, 32 (February, 1970), p. 26.

CYNTHIA'S FATHER:
I'd like to gain better understanding of my daughter's problems.

In summary, the data base obtained from the Family APGAR indicated that the subsystem of parent-child was highly dysfunctional, especially between father and daughter; however, the spouse relationship was highly functional.

5. Role changes. The parents were aware that they were no longer dealing with the conforming, compliant, prepubertal, elementary school honor student. They had a need to recognize their daughter's new role as a teenager seeking her acceptance and independence.
6. Resources. The impact of the suicide crisis was eased somewhat by the available family resources.

7. Sociocultural factors. The parents were concerned about appearances; how their upper-middle-class neighbors and friends viewed their daughter's behavior.
8. Life cycle analysis. According to the life cycle theory this family represents a combination of Rollins and Feldman's (see Figure 2-2) stages 5 and 6 (families with teenagers and families in the middle years). According to the life cycle studies, it would be expected that stages 5 and 6 would be periods of relative dysfunction. Again, it is of interest that the husband and wife interaction is at an apparent high level of function while the parent-child subsystem is at a very low level of function.

Assessment

The suicide attempt by Cynthia was a clear signal that the family needed to reach outside resources for help; the family had exceeded its coping band for crisis management. For this particular problem, Family Medical Center consultation was sought. An analysis of the family suggested the following: (1) crisis of abandonment and demoralization; (2) spouse subsystem functionally intact; (3) parent-child subsystem highly dysfunctional; and (4) identified patient (Cynthia) shows major psychosocial dysfunction.

Plan

1. Improve family member communication.
2. Initiate family therapy sessions where members will be encouraged to develop listening skills.
3. Avoid parent versus child confrontations.
4. Avoid judgmental statements.
5. Allow Cynthia an opportunity to express her feelings without fear of punishment.
6. Allow parents an opportunity to express their feelings without appearing judgmental.
7. Modification of house rules so that the psychosocial needs of all the members would be better accommodated.
8. Study further school problems (e.g., teacher, parent, physician conferences).

CONCLUSION

The integration of behavioral science into family practice presents two major challenges to the family physician: (1) the need to synthesize the care of physical with emotional problems through sensitivity to the psychosocial dimensions of the patient within the context of family and community; and (2) the need to perceive the family, not just the individual family member, as the object of care. In order to address these challenges the family physician needs a specific body of knowledge, a range of skills (including appreciation of one's potential as a therapeutic instrument), and appropriate attitudes to apply one's knowledge and skills effectively. Sections 3 and 4 of this book will focus on these areas with respect to diagnostic and treatment approaches, respectively. However, since functional and behavioral problems of individuals and their families occur in a constantly changing milieu, attention must first be directed to the issues of individual and family development, which are the subject of Section 2.

REFERENCES

1. Balint M: *The Doctor, His Patient and the Illness.* London: Pitman Medical Publishing Company, 1956
2. Mauksch HO: A social science basis for conceptualizing family health. Soc Sci Med 8:521–528, 1974
3. Engle G: The need for a new medical model: A challenge for biomedicine. Science 196:129–196, 1977
4. Drossman DA: Can the primary care physician be better trained in the psychosocial dimensions of patient care? Int J Psychiatry Med 8:169–184, 1977–78
5. Smilkstein G: A model for teaching comprehensive health care. J Med Educ 52:773–775, 1977
6. Chrisman NJ, Baker RM: Exploring the doctor-patient relationship: A socioculture pilot study in a family practice residency. J Fam Prac 7:713–719, 1978
7. Rosenstock IM: The health belief model and preventive health behavior in Becker MH (ed): The health belief model and personal health behavior. Health Educ Monogr 2:335, 1974
8. Barron F: *Creativity and Psychological Health: Origins of Personal Vitality and Creative Freedom.* New York: Van Nostrand, 1963
9. Medalie JH (ed): *Family Medicine—Principles and Applications.* Baltimore: Williams & Wilkins Co., 1978
10. Kleinman A, Eisenberg K, Good B: Culture, illness and care: Clinical lessons from anthropologic and cross-cultural research. Ann Intern Med 88:251–258, 1978
11. Kluckhohn FR: Variations in the basic values of family systems. Soc Case 39:63–72, 1958

12. Pratt L: *Family Structure and Effective Health Behavior: The Energized Family.* Boston: Houghton Mifflin Company, 1976
13. Hill R: Generic features of families under stress. Soc Cas 39:139–150, 1958
14. Haggerty RJ: "Family Crises and Intervention." In Green M, Haggerty RJ (eds): *Ambulatory Pediatrics II*, Philadelphia: W. B. Saunders Company, 1977
15. Snyder AI: Periodic marital separation and physical illness. Amer J Orthopsychiatry 48:637–643, 1978
16. Holmes TH, Masuda M: "Life Changes and Illness Susceptibility in Stressful Life Events, Their Nature and Effect." In Dohrenwend BS and Dohrenwend BP (eds): *Stressful Life Events: Their Nature and Effects.* New York: J. Wiley and Sons, 1974
17. Gunderson EKE, Rahe RR (eds): *Life Stress and Illness.* Philadelphia: Charles C. Thomas, 1974
18. Coelho GV, Hamburg DA, Adams JE (eds): *Coping and Adaptation.* New York: Basic Books, 1974
19. Miller FGW, Court SMD, Walton WS, Knox EG: *Growing Up in Newcastle Upon Tyne.* London: Oxford University Press, 1960
20. Huygen FJ: *Family Medicine—the Medical Life History of Families.* Nijmegen, The Netherlands: Decker and Vandervegt, 1978

SECTION II

Individual and Family Development

CHAPTER 3

CHILD DEVELOPMENT

GEORGE H. LOWREY

Understanding of a child's behavior and development of personality, intelligence, and cognitive abilities is inexact. Many concepts are theoretical and supported by meager experimental evidence. With this in mind, this chapter presents a review and synthesis of ideas that have proven clinically useful when evaluating children and counseling families.

Underlying the individual differences which make each human unique, there is a general pattern of development that is the same for everyone. An understanding of this sequence of stages from birth to maturity is important for both the parent and the physician. How easily or with what difficulty these stages are reached and passed depends upon many factors.[1-3]

The human organism is remarkable for its adaptability. It is extremely dependent upon social interaction for its specifically human qualities. From birth onward, there is a need for close interrelationships with protective and responsive adults in order to gain the maturity of personality for which we all strive. Personality is both genetically and environmentally influenced.

For a considerable period of time in this century the environmentalists dominated child psychology, indicating that the child's relations to family and society were most influential in shaping behavioral development. There is increasing awareness that infant and child temperament are, to a considerable extent, independent of parent-child interaction.[4] The term *temperament* designates the behavioral style, irrespective of the content, level of ability, or motivation of a particular activity. Chess and Thomas[5] state that children fall into three significant constellations of temperament, but vary widely in the degree and sharpness with which they exhibit these categories. The "easy child" is characterized by regularity, a positive mood in approach to new situations, and easy adaptability. The "difficult child" has considerable irregularity, a preponderance of withdrawal reactions to new situations, many negative mood expressions, and slow adaptability. The third type is designated "slow to warm up child." This type of child has many withdrawal responses and negative moods, mild reactions, and slow, but eventual, adaptability.

The child's temperament influences the behavior and attitudes of peers, older children, parents, and teachers. It is important for parents to recognize that all children do not react to the same stimulus in the same manner. The easy child may require so little attention as an infant that the child is actually neglected by grateful parents and later reacts with feelings of rejection. Parents of the difficult child may feel threatened and inept in their duties as caretaker. They may use pressures, appeasement, and finally punishment to accomplish toilet training, good eating habits, and avoidance of accident prone situations. Parents, like their offspring, have different temperaments and respond in varying ways to their children's behavior. It is necessary to recognize these differences when counseling parents.

FAMILY AND ENVIRONMENTAL INFLUENCES

Environmental influences begin before birth. Impaired development can result from a large number of agents including infections (especially rubella and cytomegalovirus), drugs, alcohol, and irradiation. Smoking, malnutrition, and maternal infections not transmitted to the fetus may have deleterious consequences to the developing organism.[1,6,7] Feelings or attitudes of parents toward the unborn child are of great importance in the initial acceptance and care of the pregnancy and of the newborn infant. Desire for pregnancy, economic status of the home, reactions of the father, number of siblings, the course of previous pregnancies, and the degree of nausea or other discomforts are factors having psychological influences that may carry over and influence child rearing.

A mother's acceptance of her newborn may not come immediately. Doubts and fears of her ability to assume new roles may be present.

There is increasing evidence that early and prolonged physical contact with the baby is an important element in allaying such doubts and fears.[8] Early and secure maternal-infant bonding not only gives the mother confidence, but appears to promote future behavioral benefits in the child, including improved competence in communication and language skills and more aggressive exploratory conduct. The high percentage of future behavior problems in high-risk infants may in part be due to the absence of maternal-infant bonding through the separation that results from hospitalization and isolation. The incidence of child abuse and neglect has been reduced when mothers experience close and extended contact in the neonatal period.[8, 9]

There is growing evidence that interruption or impairment of reciprocal interactions between mother and infant can lead to personality problems later in life. Nonacceptance by the parents, especially the mother, during the first 2–3 years is often associated with both withdrawn neurotic behavior and antisocial aggressiveness during later childhood and adolescence.[1, 10]

The normal child demonstrates separation anxiety and fear of strangers by 7 to 9 months. These reactions remain for about twelve months. Although overt manifestations of separation anxiety greatly decrease after the second year, some anxiety persists until at least 6 years. At that time the child can comprehend that the condition will only be temporary. Separation anxiety and its resolution reflect the infant's initial awareness of self and the beginning development of an identity as an individual. As ego strengthens, the infant learns to tolerate separation. For this reason, elective hospitalization and surgery are best delayed until after 6 years.

The impact of a new baby upon an older sibling is often apparent early in pregnancy as parents' actions and attitudes change in ways that are difficult for the sibling to comprehend. There may also be intensification in toilet training and improvement of eating techniques. Following birth, denial and rejection of the new arrival are common, as are regressions in behavior such as bed wetting or infantile conduct. The degree of this display of sibling rivalry will vary considerably depending upon age, clarity and extent of anticipatory information, and most importantly, parents' ability to demonstrate continued affection.[11]

The sexual role assimilated by the child is firmly imbedded before the fourth year when differences in sexes are clearly recognized. Sexual orientation is primarily determined by the mode of rearing. The sex roles of parents and other members of society are important in conditioning the child in his or her sex role. Children demonstrate early in their play and conversation that the male is physically stronger, more aggressive, and more punitive.

By the age of 3, information and ideas furnished and fostered by the caretakers become increasingly important to mental growth. The more extensive the education, the richer the reservoir of ideas and information. Family social differences and language abilities have enormous influence upon the intellectual performance of the child. Whether the measurement of social class is by occupation, income, or educational background, the higher the rating of the parents the stronger will be the child's school performance, I.Q. scores, and language proficiency.[1, 6, 7] Regardless of birth history, cultural or racial backgrounds, the measurable intelligence of the teenager is more clearly related to his social class than to any other factor.

COGNITIVE DEVELOPMENT

Cognition is the means by which an individual accumulates organized knowledge of his environment and self and the use of that knowledge to solve problems and modify behavior. It is a unique attribute of the human state. The initial stages of cognitive development are apparent in the infant as he recognizes and gives particular attention to familiar objects or demonstrates anticipatory behavior, such as quieting, upon approach of the mother. Piaget's theories of cognitive development are very useful in following and understanding a child's progress.[12] Table 3-1 presents an outline of a rather voluminous literature.

TABLE 3-1.   Stages of Cognitive Development

Age Span	Developmental Stage
0–2 years	Sensorimotor stage: period of exploring self and environment; early reflexes give way to purposeful actions and imitations; completely egocentric.
2–6 years	Preoperational: use of symbols for internal thought representing objects and actions; still related only to immediate experiences; much language development for social and internal use; still strongly egocentric; classification of things and actions.
6–12 years	Concrete operations: development of complex use of symbols and classification; understanding relationships (adds, subtracts, etc.); difficulty in dealing with the theoretical as opposed to the concrete.
Adolescence	Formal operations: use of the hypothetical in reasoning and methods; thinking can be propositional; extrapolation is possible; thinking may also be reflective.

MEASURING BEHAVIOR

The development examination or screening inventory is a standardized clinical procedure that can be adapted to the needs of the child. The items designated here are largely taken from the works of Gesell and his co-workers.[13] Since growth is a complex process and behavior an expression of complex interactions, interpretation must depend upon the total picture presented. A complete knowledge of growth and development is the basis for detection of abnormality. The following items represent a highly restricted and selected group of behavior patterns which can be used as reference points in screening children. It is not intended as a diagnostic examination, but as a method to alert the examiner to the need, when indicated, for further evaluation. In addition, this list may be helpful in anticipatory counseling of parents.[1, 2, 13, 14]

The predictive value of early developmental screening is not very high, especially due to the influence of socioeconomic factors during the first 3–4 years. It should be emphasized that infant tests are most useful in identifying defective development resulting from organic pathology. Few conclusions can be drawn from a single observation if any deviation from the expected is found. Such factors as emotional stability, span of attention, muscle tone and control, perceptual abilities (these include vision and hearing), fatigue, and general health status should be observed.

For screening purposes, behavior is divided into four categories, as follows:

1. Gross motor. Control of head, trunk and extremities. Motor behavior is most important in evaluating neurologic integrity.
2. Adaptive, fine motor. Manipulation and exploitation of objects. Involves the utilization of past experience in solving problems. This behavior is the most important in making judgment of intellectual potential.
3. Language. Production of sounds, words, sentences, facial and gestural expressions, and understanding the communication of others.
4. Personal-social behavior. Varies widely and depends to a large extent on culture and environment. Eating, sleep habits, toilet training, and play with others are among the items considered.

The developmental quotient is a measure of maturity and a guide to the rate of developmental progress.

$$DQ = \frac{\text{Maturity age}}{\text{Chronological age}} \times 100$$

For any one child the score may vary in each of the categories. A diagnosis does not result from a DQ score; but DQ scores can help in the complete appraisal of a child when they are supplemented with an adequate history, physical examination, and evaluation of emotional factors.

Scores may change over a period of time in a perfectly normal child. For the prematurely born infant, correction should be made from the time of conception for at least the first two years.[15, 16]

A screening examination should be accomplished in a quiet room, the mother or caretaker should be instructed not to interfere, the child should be given an opportunity to inspect the room, and test items should be introduced only when needed and then removed. All instructions should be given slowly, deliberately, and in terms the child is sure to understand. Initial tasks should be at a level easily accomplished for each category. Tasks are then presented in increasing maturational stages. The examiner should acknowledge a response as being acceptable whether or not it is correct. Although accurate evaluations, especially in personal-social items, may come from information supplied through questioning parents, actual observation of performance is preferred and has greater value in scoring.

The ages that are outlined in Table 3-2 were selected to conveniently match the usual occurrence of visits to the physician for healthy child examinations and immunization schedules. More than 66 percent of infants and children will achieve success if they come from an average North American population.

PLAY, SOCIAL BEHAVIOR, AND DISCIPLINE

Many of the important contacts between the infant or child and the environment take place through the medium of play. The pleasure this activity provides, in the presence or absence of peers and adults, serves to discharge tension and permits the exercise of imagination (sometimes in the form of "magic"). Social play, often with imaginary people, is essential for the development of the personality; it modifies egocentric concepts through exposure to the feelings and behavior of others. The child assumes many different roles in play which provide important preparation for entering adult life. Early in life, play is a useful means of decreasing dependency upon parents and serves as a catharsis of strong and sometimes frightening emotions.[12, 14]

One of the first patterns of play to develop is vocal. The obvious pleasure of repeating simple sounds appears at 3 months; babbling by 5 months. At 7 months the baby talks to his toys. Imitative play such as waving bye-bye or pat-a-cake appears between 9 and 11 months, at

TABLE 3-2. Screening Inventory

	Gross Motor	Adaptive, Fine Motor	Personal-Social	Language
2–4 Weeks	1. Asymmetric tonic neck reflex position 2. Prone, turns head 3. Head sags if held sitting	1. Regards object in line of vision 2. Follows to midline 3. Hands fisted 4. Drops toys immediately	1. Small throaty noises 2. Vague regard	1. Sight or sound stimulus diminishes activity 2. Stares at surroundings
2 Months	1. Mixed posture-asymmetric and symmetric 2. Prone, lifts head recurrently 3. Head bobs erect if held sitting	1. Delayed regard of toy held in midline 2. Follows past midline 3. Hands loosely fisted, sometimes open 4. Holds toys briefly	1. Single vowel sounds "o, e, u" 2. Alert response to voice or face	1. Beginning smile 2. Eyes follow moving face
3 Months	1. Symmetric posture dominates 2. Prone, lifts head sustained 3. Head briefly held erect if sitting	1. Prompt regard of toy held in midline 2. Follows toy 180° with eye and head movement 3. Hands open most of time 4. Holds toy sustained	1. Coo and chuckle 2. Social vocal responses	1. Looks at examiner predominately 2. Regards own hands 3. Pulls and pokes at clothing

37

TABLE 3-2. Cont.

	Gross Motor	Adaptive, Fine Motor	Personal-Social	Language
4 Months	1. Symmetric posture predominates 2. Prone, lifts head to 90°, may push chart off table 3. Head steadily erect if sitting	1. Waves arms, moves body at sight of toy 2. Regards toy in hand 3. Takes toy to mouth 4. Brings hands to midline and plays with fingers	1. Laughs aloud 2. Excites, wiggles, breathes rapidly in play	1. Spontaneous social smile 2. Anticipates food on sight
6 Months	1. Can roll over 2. Supports most of weight if held standing 3. May sit by leaning on hands if put in position	1. Reaches for and grasps toy, brings to mouth 2. Can recover toy dropped if in reach 3. Crude transfer of toy from hand to hand 4. Bangs toy up and down if sitting	1. Squeals, grunts and growls 2. Imitates some sounds "ma-ma, da-da" 3. Repeats vowel sound in series "o-o-o" etc.	1. Recognizes difference of family and strangers 2. Talks to mirror image and pats it with hands
9 Months	1. Can sit erect for 5-10 minutes or longer 2. Crawls 3. Stands with only slight support 4. May pull self to standing position	1. Can release grasp to accept another toy 2. Explores with index finger 3. Pincer grasp 4. Searches for hidden object	1. Says and means "ma-ma" and "da-da" 2. Knows own name 3. Can imitate sounds, e.g. cough	1. Feeds self finger foods 2. May play a nursery trick: wave bye-bye, pat-a-cake, etc.

Age	Motor	Adaptive	Language	Personal-Social
12 Months	1. Walks with one hand held or alone 2. Stands alone 3. Cruises (walks using stationary objects for support)	1. Puts cube in cup after demonstration 2. Dangles toy by string 3. Pincer grasp refined 4. Attempts to build cube tower	1. Two or three words plus "ma-ma" and "da-da" with proper meaning 2. Places toy in examiner's hand	1. Helps in dressing 2. Explores surrounding
18 Months	1. Climbs into adult chair 2. Walks upstairs with stationary support 3. Rarely falls with walking	1. Builds tower of three or more cubes 2. Dumps raisins out of bottle 3. Imitates crayon stroke on paper 4. Scribbles spontaneously	1. Has ten words 2. Can follow at least one verbal direction, e.g., take ball to mother, put it on the table, etc. 3. On request points to parts of body: eyes, nose, hair (at least one)	1. Feeds self with spoon, messy 2. Pulls string toy 3. Hugs doll or stuffed animal
2 Years	1. Runs well 2. Walks up and down stairs with no support 3. Kicks large ball	1. Builds tower of six or more cubes 2. Turns pages of book singly 3. Imitates crayon vertical and circular strokes	1. Uses pronouns (not always grammatical) 2. Two and three word sentences 3. Follows four directions with ball 4. Can point to several parts of body	1. Pulls on simple garment 2. Plays with domestic mimicry
3 Years	1. Balances on one foot for at least one second 2. Alternates feet going upstairs 3. Rides tricycle using pedals	1. Builds tower of nine or more cubes 2. Imitates three cube bridge 3. Copies circle	1. Uses plurals 2. Gives sex and full name 3. Names eight pictures correctly (cup, house, dog, cat, book, man)	1. Feeds self well 2. Puts on shoes 3. Understands taking turns

TABLE 3-2. Cont.

	Gross Motor	Adaptive, Fine Motor	Personal-Social	Language
4 Years	1. Does broad jump 2. Alternates feet going downstairs 3. Can throw ball overhead	1. Counts three objects correctly 2. Draws person with two or three parts 3. Copies cross 4. Picks longer of two lines	1. Obeys five prepositions: on, under, in front, in back, beside 2. Names primary colors 3. Comprehends cold, hungry, tired	1. Undresses without assistance 2. Washes and dries face and hands
5 Years	1. Stands on one foot more than eight seconds 2. Catches bounced tennis ball	1. Counts ten objects correctly 2. Draws person with body, head, extremities 3. Copies square	1. Names penny, nickel, dime 2. Knows four or more colors 3. Uses all parts of speech	1. Dresses without assistance 2. Bossy and critical
6 Years	1. Hops on one foot 2. Walks backward heel-toe on line 3. Throws ball accurately	1. Adds and subtracts within five 2. Draws person with more detail, fingers, clothing, etc. 3. Copies diamond	1. Defines words by function or content, house is to live in 2. Can tell familiar story 3. Prints full name	1. Ties shoelaces 2. Knows difference between A.M. and P.M. 3. Can repeat eight word sentence

which time the baby can accomplish a broad spectrum of facial expressions. By 14–15 months play includes activity with a favorite doll or stuffed toy which also may be used to allay fears when going to bed. At this time there is considerable conversation and the beginning of role taking with toys. This is further elaborated at 2 years by the child assuming the role of the parent. Previously undirected play merges into practice play with evident objectives. The child repeats play because of enjoyment with the pleasantly familiar. Repetition provides a means to gain confidence and self-assurance, thereby developing the ego. The child watches, listens, and imitates. Repetition and imitation constitute important aspects of play throughout life.

The pleasures of play and the opposing influence of discipline can lead to some anxieties. Most children can cope with these disturbing emotions and the desire to explore is not destroyed. One method of coping with frustrations and anger is by acting out or dramatizing feelings through symbolic play. A doll may be spanked or scolded for bad behavior. In the fantasy of play one can do many things forbidden or frightening in real-life situations.

At 3 years, the average child is sufficiently mature to enter into cooperative play. This involves sharing and taking turns. The 4 year old is sufficiently self-assured to be argumentative, boastful, and aggressive. Verbal profanity is sometimes practiced. Much of this results from the desire to experience new actions or words, as well as being a test of parental reaction. At this age, the first indications of a conscience and of self-criticism are observed.

Play in the early school years is characterized by the need of conformity and tends to be very ritualistic. Much of play at any age involves the acquisition of skills and leads to further self-confidence as the child gains in stature with peers. By 7 or 8 segregation of the sexes in play becomes a factor in the choice of playmates.

The child learns and gains competence by experimenting. Parents need to be supportive without fostering excessive dependence or inhibiting the development of skills. Parents who are aware of the developmental continuum experienced by all children are better able to cope with behavior problems when they arise. Mothers, fathers, and other caretakers need to manage children in terms of their present capabilities, their cultural heritage, and anticipation of developmental requirements. The aim is to achieve security and independence that is commensurate with the child's level of development.

To become an accepted member of the community, children need to acquire a set of socially desirable traits. Firm but reasonable expectations of behavior are effective in guiding children. Without guidelines and limits that are set and consistently followed by parents, the infant and child feel lost, helpless, and unloved. When discipline is necessary, the child must understand the reason for it. Its administration should not be unduly delayed beyond the event which necessitated it. Discipline which is consistent, firm, and does not ask the impossible is seldom unsuccessful. If it is administered in an unpredictable fit of anger and threatens the withdrawal of parental love, it is poorly accepted and creates unnecessary fear and anxiety. One can explain to the child that feelings of anger or frustration are understandable, but the behavior was unacceptable. The explanation can assure the child of continued affection. Punishment should never be used as a means of retribution by one parent or another.

THE ADOLESCENT

Adolescence is that period of life associated with accelerated growth in both height and weight, the maturation of sexual characteristics and functions, and a subsequent, rapid deceleration of growth that terminates in the fusion of the epiphyses and metaphyses. It is a period of transition from childhood to adulthood. It has no sharp end points, either at the beginning or at the end, and lasts almost a decade. There is considerable variability in the chronologic ages at which these events occur.

Puberty refers to that time when sexual reproduction is possible. Common law and most legal statutes refer to the word in that manner. Menarche is often used as the indicator of puberty, though ovulation and the ability to reproduce is often not present for a year or two after menarche. The beginning of adolescence, puberty, and cessation of growth occurs in girls about two years earlier than in boys. As indicated, however, there is great variation in the chronological age at which each of these events occur. For example, in the United States the average age of menarche is just under 13 years, but approximately 14 percent of girls will have their first menstrual period before their twelfth birthday, 10 percent after their fourteenth birthday.[1, 17]

In addition to the dramatic changes in growth and sexual maturation, the rise in androgenic hormones is responsible for the appearance of acne. It is worth remembering that acne is a universal problem in this age group and its course or severity provokes much anxiety and sometimes unpredictable behavior, e.g., food fads or asceticism.

The last two decades have brought about decided changes in the psycho-social patterning of adolescent development. Among these changes is the disappearance of the multigenerational and geographically stable family. An increasing number of children are being raised by a single parent. The great increase in numbers of teenagers, beginning in the 1950s, placed considerable pressure on the secondary schools. This development, combined with a long compulsory education requirement, forced children into more narrowly defined age groups with increasing isolation. World and regional armed conflicts, cold wars, social and racial inequalities, and dishonesty in government have led to disillusionment and rejection of ideas and opinions from parents and other adults. The atmosphere of permissiveness in rearing children from 1940 to 1970 has led to a weakening of young peoples' regard for all kinds of discipline. All of these factors have affected the psycho-social development of adolescents.

Other factors which have played a lesser part in influencing adolescent attitudes include religious and technologic changes. In contrast to past generations, religion has not assumed a strong role in leadership for youth. Improved means of communication, especially television, have permitted a great dissemination of information, both good and bad, resulting in a false sense of superior knowledge and sophistication. Finally, the rapid technologic progress over the last two to three decades, which seemed to promise solutions for many social, economic, and educational problems, has failed to accomplish its goals. This has led to further disillusionment among young men and women regarding career choices.

These disappointments and isolation have resulted in the formation of an adolescent peer society as a semi-autonomous social world with its own set of values. Peers, rather than parents or other adults, are looked to as the model for dress, entertainment, and life style. Peer group association is prized above all other associations. Increasing numbers of young people leave the mainstream of life, at least temporarily, in an attempt to resolve the identity crisis. Although the degree of withdrawal may depend upon previous intra-family relationships, even the most conforming children seek some independence from their parents.[17]

All adolescents at some time, and in various ways, will solve their own identity crisis in order to enter and adjust to the adult world. This is a normative stage in the human life cycle. Youth is faced with the decision of which choices to follow in his or her sexual, social, and occupational roles as an adult. A few will become members of a religious group, a radical political party, an anarchist group, or a cult movement. A few will become drifters and drop outs perhaps relying on drugs to find the answers.

Although sexual education begins early in childhood, often with the arrival of a sibling, many adolescents have extremely limited knowledge of important aspects of how and when conception occurs. Unfortunately, many hold the opinion that improved methods of contraception and treatments for veneral diseases have removed the hazards of acting out sexual impulses. In the United States one-fifth of all pregnancies occur in women under 19 years of age, and half of these in girls under 17.

More than two-thirds of these pregnancies are conceived out of wedlock. Many reasons are given for the pregnancies, including: a way to punish parents, a means to keep a boyfriend, "to prove I'm grown up," and as a method to obtain something that will return and show affection and love. But by far the most common reason is ignorance of the consequences of sexual intercourse or the means to prevent those consequences.[1, 17]

Sexual activity before marriage is still largely socially and religiously forbidden. This often leads to feelings of guilt that unfortunately may be retained well into adult life by the individual. Many parents still look upon most sexual activity as pleasant and necessary but somehow sinful. Even though the phenomena of sexuality is more openly discussed by today's youth, sources of information are frequently inadequate. This is especially so if the source of information is peers. However, parents often are in need of education themselves and they may be overly judgmental in their opinions. It has been repeatedly stressed that the child's experience of parents' attitudes and behavior is an extremely important element in that child's final sexual adjustment.

For the adolescent, the inability to choose an occupational identity is very disturbing. Pressures to make such a decision come from family, peers, the expectations of the society, and the pressure of one's own desires concerning the future. Limitations on accomplishments result from these pressures, socioeconomic status, level of intelligence, various achievements of the past, and whether previous achievements have resulted in satisfaction or frustration. The tendency of the adolescent who is continually faced with failure as judged by the conventions of society or parental attitudes, is to react with aggressive rebellion. This leads to further difficulties and a vicious cycle can result. A realistic philosophy or goal in life is needed, which furnishes the adolescent with motivation to accomplish the best of which he or she is capable.

Parents should recognize and accept changing relationships between themselves and their children. This amounts to a steadily growing equality. Parents and educators must realize that social, economic, and moral values change with each generation. The adult must serve as an experienced guide who has greater information and the advantage in most spheres of mature ability. At the same time, there must be an equality of human dignity and personal integrity between the adult and child. The parents must help the adolescent complete emancipation by allowing and encouraging reasonable independence. Often parents find it disturbing and difficult to accept their children's growing discreditation. If such parents have few interests outside the family and their own marital life has been unfulfilled, they may resort to punitive and derogatory attacks on the child. Such reactions result in further discords and increased separation.

REACTIONS TO ILLNESS

The infant reacts to illness by a variety of responses that involve many body systems. Crying, refusing to eat, vomiting, and resisting sleep are examples. Some of these responses may constitute an inherent part of the illness itself, but some do not.

For the child, hospitalization not only means separation from family and friends, but a great many other changes, all anxiety producing. There is more or less confinement to bed or room; the illness itself or diagnostic and therapeutic procedures cause discomfort or pain; the food is different; hospital attire does not resemble what is worn at home, even to bed; toileting facilities are strange or far removed, or the use of a bedpan is required; most loved and familiar objects are not available; and, finally, people who perform tasks are mostly strangers. How could such an experience be anything but fear producing?

If hospitalization is necessary, separation from parents becomes the major problem. Separation in these circumstances may also be associated with many kinds of discomfort or pain. Stress for the child will be equaled by stress for the parents. When possible, rooming-in arrangements for parents should be provided. Lacking such accommodations, prolonged visits and as many parenting functions as possible should be permitted. Frequent visits with the physician are comforting and reassuring.[18]

For the older child, preparation for hospitalization through education of both child and parents should be undertaken when possible. A well-illustrated book or pamphlet prepared for the child's level of development can be helpful in allaying some anxieties. A visit to the hospital is a valuable technique. Familiar toys or books indicate there has not been total abandonment. Personnel involved with the child's care should be aware that all that is seen and heard is taken quite literally. Throughout the preschool period the child thinks of illness, taking medicine, and healing as a kind of fantasy invloving some good and bad magic. These ideas need to be appreciated and must not be dismissed or ignored as being unreasonable.

The school age child can understand some of the basic aspects of illness and can reason about cause and effect. There is still some retention of the fantasy or magical approach for explaining points that are too complex or not readily available to the senses. When possible, procedures and instruments that are to be used should be shown or explained, being careful to use language that is simple and direct.

For the adolescent, the emotional impact of serious illness or injury may be as disabling as the condition itself. An understanding of coping methods used by this age group will enhance the physician's ability to manage the situation. Destructive denial, regression, and even panic are possible reactions. These can be blunted and converted to useful compensation and intellectualization by a sympathetic health team. Recognition of the need for independence and self-determination is important, as is concern about the integrity of the body image. To aid the hospitalized adolescent, the ward setting should encourage as much independence as possible, yet provide a degree of privacy. The patient should be encouraged to participate in decisions about his or her care; to pursue as much self-management as possible; to engage in establishing a peer group on the ward; and to continue school education. The staff should recognize and praise, when appropriate, the adolescent's courage in a difficult situation.[19]

A few comments about the issues of death and dying with children are appropriate. Before 3 or 4, the child has little or no concept of death and does not differentiate it from sleep. Older preschoolers have usually had some experience with death through the loss of a pet or relative. Even so, they generally conceive of death as being reversible. This is substantiated by stories, television, and comics where there is often a reappearance of persons who have died.

The school age child is usually more concerned with bodily harm than the abstract concept of death. Death is considered a very prolonged sleep and prompts such questions as "What happens when they put him in the ground?" and "Who does he play with when he dies?" or "Doesn't he ever get hungry?" There may also be the fantasy of death as a kind of monster that comes in the night to claim its victims.

The adolescent perceives death for the first time as an irreversible process. This brings forth thoughts about the meaning of life in general and the reason for existence. The fear of dying alone is perhaps stronger than any other.

A child is influenced by the family's attitudes and religious beliefs. There are many morally and ethically correct ways to meet the questions and anxieties of the patient and the family. Most importantly the physician listens and observes the levels of understanding that exist and responds accordingly. It is important to absolve the parents from blame; not only by making such a statement, but also by giving the reason why the statement is true. Expressions of sorrow by the physician and other members of the health team are very supportive to parents. The availability of the physician to answer questions to the grieving parents and to share their sorrow is most important.

CONCLUSIONS

Many attempts have been made to formulate the basic needs of childhood whose fulfillment would satisfy a normal emotional development. The following list may not be complete, but recognition of these factors is of utmost importance in our attempt to facilitate the development of the happy and well-adjusted child.

1. Security. Feeling of belonging to family and social groups. The child thrives on love, but also needs firm and kindly guidance. Too permissive an approach leads to a feeling of abandonment and insecurity.
2. Adaptability. Learning to live in the world as it is. This means facing reality and conforming with the group. It does not mean unquestioned acquiescence to the environment.
3. Freedom. Expression of one's individuality. A child should be allowed to fantasize, to daydream, and to use imagination. Guidance does not imply constant adult direction or advice.
4. Achievement of success. Allowing the child considerable self-expression often leads to self-identification of outstanding capabilities. Praise on the part of parents should always be commensurate with the task achieved. Nothing builds the ego as much as well-earned success and praise by peers and parents.

REFERENCES

1. Lowrey GH: *Growth and Development of Children.* Chicago: Year Book Medical Publishers, Inc., 1978
2. Senn MJE and Solnit AJ: *Problems in Child Behavior and Development.* Philadelphia: Lea and Febiger, 1968
3. Schulte FJ: "The Neurological Development of the Neonate." In Davis JA, and Dobbin J (eds): *Scientific Foundations of Paediatrics.* Philadelphia: W. B. Saunders Co., 1974
4. Thomas A, Chess S, and Birch H: *Temperament and Behavioral Disorders in Children.* New York: University Press, 1968
5. Thomas A and Chess S: *Temperament and Development.* New York: Brunner-Mazel, 1977.
6. Chase HP and Martin HP: Undernutrition and child development. N Eng J Med 282:933, 1970
7. Dobbing J and Sands J: Vulnerability of developing brain; IX: The effect of nutritional growth retardation on the timing of the brain growth spurt. Biol Neonate 19:363, 1971
8. Klaus MH and Kennell JH: *Maternal-Infant Bonding.* St. Louis: C. V. Mosby Co., 1976
9. O'Connor SM, Vietze PM, Hopkins JB and Altemeir WA: Postpartum extended maternal-infant contact: Subsequent mothering and child health. Pediatr Res 11:380, 1977
10. Ainsworth MDS: The development of infant-mother attachment. *Rev Child Develop Res* 3:1, 1973
11. Bakwin H and Bakwin RM: *Behavior Disorders in Children.* 4th ed. Philadelphia: W. B. Saunders Co., 1972
12. Piaget J: *The Psychology of the Child.* New York: Basic Books, Inc., 1969
13. Knoblock H and Pasamanick B (eds): *Developmental Diagnosis.* 3rd ed. New York: Harper and Row Publishers, Inc., 1975

14. Erikson EH: *Childhood and Society.* 2nd ed. New York: W. W. Norton, 1963
15. Saint-Anne Dargassies S: Long term neurological follow-up study of 286 truly premature infants. Develop Med Child Neurol 19:462, 1977
16. Lubchenco, LO: *The High Risk Infant.* Philadelphia: W. B. Saunders Co., 1976
17. Erikson EH: *Identity, Youth and Crisis.* New York: W. W. Norton, 1968
18. Kenny TJ: The hospitalized child. Pediatr Clin North America, 22583, 1975
19. Hofmann AD: The impact of illness in adolescence and coping behavior. Acta Paediatr Scand (Suppl), 256:29, 1975

CHAPTER 4

ADULT DEVELOPMENT

THOMAS L. LEAMAN

Children tend to see themselves as always changing; bigger than last year, able and allowed to do more things than last year, but not as big as some other children and not able to do many of the things they want to do. They see adults as having grown up, having arrived. Often we adults tend to see each other as being in relatively stable situations, not changing much from year to year. At class reunions we tend to expect to find people as we left them ten or twenty years ago. There seems, however, a tendency for us to see our selves in constant change; growing intellectually, maturing emotionally, changing spiritually, or struggling physically.

Family physicians, from a perspective of several decades of close personal contact with the same people, recognize that most people's lives are crowded with crises and changes. They see few adults in whom there are not major personal changes in the recent past, present, or impending future. Rarely does a family, or even an individual, spend five years without internal and external major changes in their personal milieu.

Figures 4-1 and 4-2 are Currier and Ives prints indicating the artists' conception of the stages of man and the stages of woman. It is especially interesting that there is no middle-aged plateau, the stages are quite

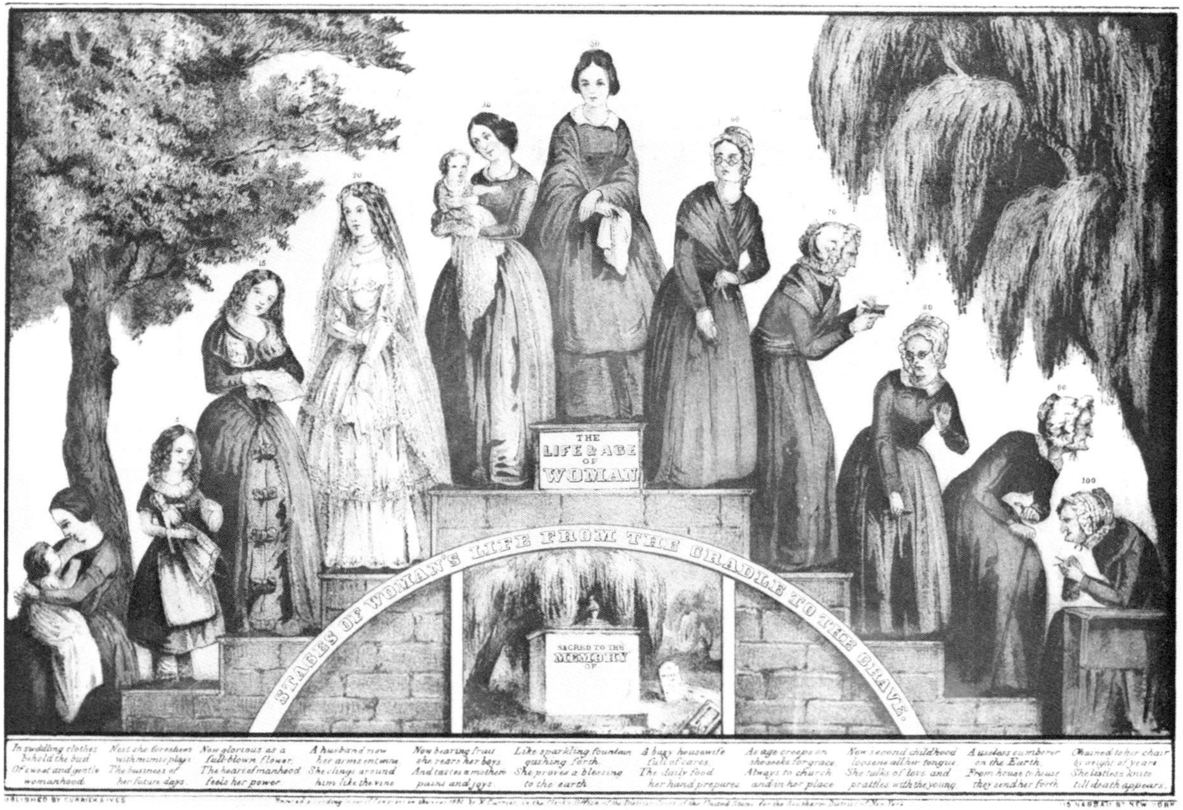

FIGURE 4-1. An early American view of the stages of life in woman.

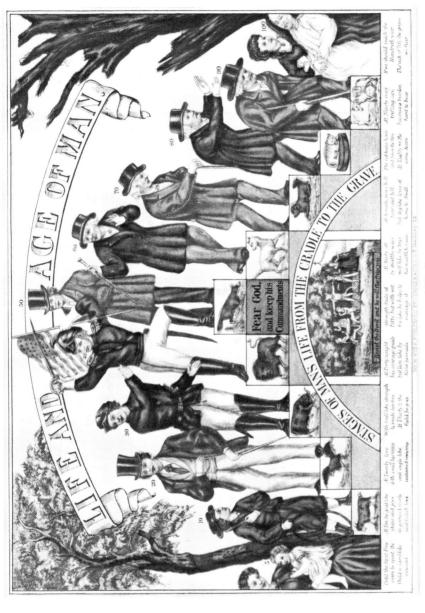

FIGURE 4-2. An early American view of the stages of life in man.

51

symmetrical and quite similar. Now, nearly two centuries later, is there much difference in our understanding of the adult developmental process? There do appear to be several significant changes in perception. The summit seems to have shifted somewhat to the right for most individuals. There is also greater recognition of individual variability.

We are, as individuals, extremely complex; we may be growing in some areas but are declining in others. There are not two with identical patterns. A model, such as the one depicted in Figures 2-1 and 2-2, may be of interest in understanding groups, but can never be applied to an individual. There is a growing realization that our own stimuli and motivation, and our milieu, can exert great influence on our individual patterns. The model seems to show a picture of "what happens to us" in a passive way; yet much of what happens to us is under our direct influence, if not control. Certainly this is applicable in our emotional, spiritual, and intellectual development. We also have considerable influence over physical changes when it is considered that a high proportion of ailments are self inflicted through intemperate habits, accidents, poor nutrition, and failure to use known health maintenance mechanisms.

Every family physician knows the value of helping an individual or family plan for major life changes such as retirement, marriage, birth, and death. Planning for the future helps us to understand ourselves and our patients. Thus, it is vital that we learn as much as possible about adult growth and development.

The purpose of this chapter is to survey the area of adult development from early adulthood through old age. Developmental changes, predictable life crises, and possible resources for coping with these alterations will be considered. The objectives for us, as health care providers, are:

1. To understand patients as they are becoming.
2. To help patients prepare for change and to understand the predictability and inevitability of some changes.
3. To help patients appreciate the kinds of changes that are normal versus abnormal.
4. To help patients see opportunities arising from change.
5. To understand ourselves as adults.

STAGES OF ADULTHOOD

> *For the normal adult, going through this period is like heading west of Denver where there are few plateaus.*
>
> John P. Vanderpool

TABLE 4-1.   The Six Stages of Adulthood*

Stage	Age Range
1. Leaving Home for Real	18 years to 20/25 years
2. Early Adulthood	20/25 years to 30/35 years
3. Midlife Crises	35 years to 40/45 years
4. Middle Adulthood	40/45 years to 60 years
5. Preparation for Retirement	60 years to 65 years
6. Advanced Adulthood	65 years to death

* Vanderpool JP: New visions of adulthood. Cont Ed 7:94–109, 1977

Many classifications have been developed to try to describe the different phases of adulthood. Since there are no distinct boundaries or definitive criteria; and since there is wide variation among individuals and groups, any such statement can only provide a framework. However, it is helpful to use such a framework to attempt to understand ourselves and our patients. The six stages of adulthood as described by Vanderpool (Table 4-1) seem most appropriate for purposes of this chapter. It is designed to describe American adults. Vanderpool[1] notes that in this staging there appear to be two kinds of alternate life stages: (1) those characterized by change and transition; and (2) those characterized by relative developmental stability. Stages I, III, V are periods of transition while alternating stages are times of relative stability.

Leaving Home for Real

This is the period when the young adult actually moves out of home. Frequently there are many temporary moves before it becomes for real. It is a time of college, of beginning a career, of military services, often of living together or marriage. It is a time of frequent personal struggles and many active changes—personal, sexual, occupational, educational, and philosophical. It is also a time of experimenting with new lifestyles, of travel, and of trying new locations.

The principal psychological tasks, as pointed out by Vanderpool, are "establishing one's own identity, learning to develop intimacy with others, and separating from one's family." The problem of who am I? is acute and must be addressed before the other two. Failure or delay often leads to a sense of alienation and depression. This developmental issue should be recognized by the physician and the family as early as possible and support should be provided where appropriate.

This is an age of good general health except for those impediments that are self inflicted through drugs, alcohol, accidents, and anxiety/depression. Failure in learning to develop intimacy with others and/or separating from one's own family leads to multiple personal and social problems and to a high rate of divorce.

The family physician's challenge, with patients in this age group, is to recognize and help patients recognize their needs and hazards and identify various sources of support. The symptoms that may arise during this period of turmoil may not be the symptoms which patients traditionally take to physicians.

Early Adulthood

By this time most young adults will have worked out some acceptable answer to the question of who they are, they will have begun to develop intimacy with others, and they will have made a successful and necessary separation from their previous family. They are now ready to begin a family of their own. Most young adults marry or form a one-to-one relationship outside of marriage. This period is accompanied by a combination of excitement over possibilities and self-assurance over ability to cope, with some anxieties that things might not work out as hoped, or an inability to cope. In general, confidence seems to far outweigh caution.

The major changes involve both personal life and career. Finding a spouse or a significantly intimate other can help in the establishment of personal growth, stability, and confidence. Finding mentors in the business or professional world is also important.

This is usually an age of good general physical health, although stress-related illnesses may begin to appear at this time. The family physician's task is to be sensitive to such possibilities and to devise means of remaining in touch with patients during this stage. As in the previous stage, the symptoms that arise may not be those that suggest a visit to the physician.

Mid-Life Crisis

For some individuals, this time period represents a time of planned and deliberate change as a result of gradual realization of the limitations of one's own life. However, for many, perhaps most, there is a very real crisis. The individual comes rather suddenly to grips with his or her mortality, there is a limited time left to fulfill hopes and dreams, and there is a "downside" to life. If one wishes to change jobs or spouses now is the time—what employer or spouse will want someone older?

Vanderpool points out that a crisis might be triggered by some specific event, either one of major import or seemingly trivial, e.g., "being beaten in a tennis game by one's son; looking in a mirror and noting wrinkles; or the fact that everything has dropped an inch lower; feeling chronically depressed or bored; having the last child leave for school; having a coronary; agonizing over the death of a parent, etc." He points out that this crisis state usually has three phases: shock/impact, recoil/turmoil, and resolution. Those who are able to recognize a crisis, meet it, and find a satisfactory resolution often emerge with significant changes in their life, and an improved sense of personal confidence. In the initial stages of shock/impact, there is much soul searching, and grief over things lost or dreams unachieved. This phase often leads to depression, which may be followed by the formulation of new plans, an altered life style, or a search for a career change.

Gail Sheehy[2] identifies several factors that may lead to a crisis at this age in women, including sending the last child off to school or returning to the working world. Statistically, it is a time when a woman is most likely to have an affair, when most divorced women are likely to marry, and when reproduction becomes ill-advised.

The health hazards of this age are more numerous and they present opportunities for primary care physicians, in prevention and treatment. Stress-related ailments are seen with increasing frequency. The death rate for men, especially related to cardiovascular disease, is also increased. Alcoholism and drug abuse (particularly of tranquilizers) is high. Family conflicts and psychosocial problems are prominent and the potential for drastic outcomes is high. Yet, the opportunities for prevention and active intervention by family physicians are also high. Most adults by this time have formed patient-doctor relationships. The patient-doctor relationship can form the base for increasing insight and active support.

The mid-life crisis, like all other stages, is a time of infinite variation from person to person. Barbara Fried[3] in her epilogue to *The Middle-Age Crisis* says:

> It goes without saying that the external details of any individual real life crisis will not conform at all or even in most respects to the simplified and abstracted generalizations used to illustrate the crisis here. Each of us is himself as well as Everyman, and our unique histories and personal endowments shape what we do and how we feel and react. At the same time, though, it is necessary to keep in

mind that our individual responses and special cases, although they make all the difference in the world to us, are actually only slight variations within the broad context of a life long and universal process of development and growth. We may sail more or less close to the winds of change during the crisis years, but essentially we're all in the same boat.

Middle Adulthood

For those who have successfully resolved the issues of the previous stage, this may be a period of great stability and productivity. The individual has demonstrated that crises can be handled and faces the day-to-day problems with renewed confidence. The major kinds of problems which likely need to be faced are the death of a parent, increasing career responsibility, and children in late teenage and early adult years. The marriage is likely to have developed a firmer aspect, being a supporting factor rather than contributing to the problems of living.

For the individual or couple who have not satisfactorily resolved their aging, or have not faced it, middle age may be a continuation of the previous crisis or a time of turning inward to a dull, day-to-day, self-centered existence. For men and women in careers, this is likely to be the time of peak productivity, opportunity for creativity, and maximum responsibility. There is a grave danger of the "empty nest" syndrome, the woman who has invested her whole sense of purpose in the production and rearing of children, and whose children have now left, may feel a sense of worthlessness. This may be compounded by the menopausal syndrome.

The health problems of this age begin to become increasingly frequent and more apparent. Chronic diseases begin frequently at this period, especially arthritis, cardiovascular disease, obesity, and diabetes. There is further increase in the male death rate and frequent psychological changes concurrent with all of these events. Perhaps even more than in earlier years, since most marriages enter a new stage of stability and interdependence, these health problems produce profound effects on the other partner. A sensitive physician will always search for these effects in order to provide support in coping.

Preparation for Retirement

Often at the time of a person's peak productivity and greatest responsibility, thought must be given to a forced retirement, usually at age 65. This also is a period of transition that differs from other transitions in preparation for a decrease in activities rather than an increase.

Preparations require development of new interests, or of old interests in a new way, financial rearrangements, and new adjustments within the marriage. Preparations by the noncareer spouse include adjustment to having the partner (usually him in our present culture, but this may be changing) at home all day. Failure to make preparations can lead to frustration, boredom, a sense of worthlessness, and resultant depression.

The task of the family physician at this stage is to help raise the awareness of the couple to the need for such preparations. While adults know for fifty years that retirement is coming, it is surprising how frequently the need for preparation is ignored or denied. Other tasks for the physician at this time include sensitivities to the possibilities of depression (there is a higher suicide rate for men at this time), continued care of multiple chronic disease problems, and the need to help individuals learn to live within declining physical capabilities.

Advanced Adulthood

Vanderpool in his description of stages has divided this group into two sub-groups: "a younger group that is healthy and vigorous and the old, old who are plagued by disability and disease." The younger of the two is likely to be active in social and political affairs and wield considerable power. The "old, old" group is relatively helpless and/or withdrawn from the outside world. There are more women than men who survive to this stage. As a total group this population over 65 has now reached 22 million. It is expected that within the decade this group will increase by another 5 million.

Erikson lists the developmental crisis at this age to be that of integrity versus despair.[4] The person who can look with satisfaction on life or at least accept it as the best he/she could do under the circumstances, and would probably do it all over again, has reached a degree of integrity. Those who cannot look beyond and wish it were different or wish they had done something else suffer from despair.

Vanderpool points out that there is a danger in stereotyping old people as "all the same," a form of prejudice which he calls "agism." This may be a reflection, he states, of the fear by each of us of growing old. The physician has the opportunity to understand patients' sensitivities in intimate ways and needs to guard against this prejudice. Declining hearing, dimmed vision, dulled perception, faltering memory may all lead to difficulties in communication. At the same time there is a greater need for understanding of feelings, efforts to communicate, struggles to cope, and appreciation of perspective. Simple openness and blunt honesty is in order. In most patients such communication is deeply appreciated and painful emotions may be tempered by a sense of humor.

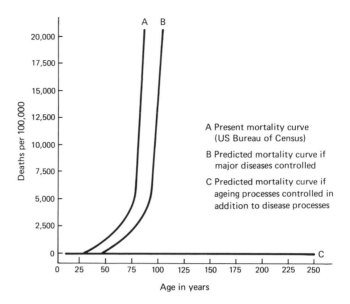

FIGURE 4-3.   Actual and predicted mortality curves. This figure compares the mortality curve in the US (curve A) with what could be predicted if all major diseases were conquered but no change was made in the aging problem itself (curve B), and if the factors leading to aging were also brought under control (curve C). It is obvious that the only way to make a material increase in longevity is to control aging processes themselves (Soddy K & Kidson MC: Men in Middle Life. Philadelphia: J. B. Lippincott Company, 1967, p. 68).

Aging is a process of slowing and gradual reduction in functioning. It must be understood as separate from disease processes, which may be more amenable to treatment. It is important to realize that the maximum length of human life has probably not altered for many centuries. The fact that many more persons approach the maximum period of life (around 100 years) is attributable to the overcoming of many diseases or the delaying of their effects. Figure 4-3 demonstrates the overall outcome of mankind's efforts to lengthen life by conquering disease and his total ineffectiveness in lengthening the life span. Visits to physicians increase rapidly at this age group as organic and functional disease and the problems inherent in the aging process increase. Cardiovascular diseases are the most common, followed, or accompanied, by arthritis, cancer, accidents related to the effects of aging, diabetes, and various lung diseases. Ailments of the sensory organs are also increasingly prominent and problematic.

Psychological and social problems increase and paranoid thinking becomes a more common problem. While the aged person usually has learned to cope more philosophically than younger persons with important losses, the necessity for coping with multiple personal losses may become exceedingly difficult; loss of friends, home, independence, sufficient income, and especially spouse and health. Social problems are common and include loneliness, the need for being cared for by others, loss of real communication, exploitation, and the fear of exploitation.

The tasks for physicians have been described throughout this discussion. Perhaps the greatest opportunity is for the physician to understand each patient as an individual, to help others understand them as individuals, and to accept them as members of a continuum rather than a group apart.

DEVELOPMENTAL CHANGES

Any discussion of physical changes in adult development must be prefaced by an understanding that only the roughest of generalizations is possible and that there are great individual differences and numerous individual patterns. In attempting to understand an individual, it is helpful to have a general knowledge of both the normative and the range of variations. In this brief overview, we will touch on topics of particular interest with no attempt at a comprehensive study of possibilities.

Physical Changes

While adulthood is a period of relative physical stability, there is a constant series of changes taking place. They are generally subtle, regressive, and negative. Some changes begin at the earliest stage of adulthood, others have their onset during middle age. Even though some physical changes do begin early, adulthood is generally the time of full growth and development in strength, coordination, health, efficiency, and endurance.[5] This period generally lasts 20 to 30 years; noticeable changes begin, on an average, about the age of 50.

Physical size and strength usually reach a maximum between the ages of 25 and 30. However, this obvious information is of little value because of the great individual variation. Of much more value in the understanding of the individual is that person's self-perception. Troll has stated, "as a rule those people who derive their feelings of worth from their bodies (e.g. strong men, athletes, or beautiful women) are likely to be more sensitive to decreases in physical attributes than those who have other ways of assessing their value."[5]

There is a demonstrable decline in manual dexterity in the adult years; but because of other factors including training, skills and motivation, the decline in manual dexterity is not generally paralleled by a decrease in job performance (e.g., the musician whose performance depends on finger skills).

While it is common experience that chronological age may vary markedly from functional age, no means has yet been accepted for a different kind of measurement. Retirement and various legal status changes are based on chronological age. Yet, it would seem that resources now exist, through psychological, biological and performance testing, to develop some acceptable means for assessing functional level, much as developmental testing is performed in infants. It would not require great precision to be more accurate than currently accepted chronological age assessment!

Sensory Perceptions

Some aging changes in the eye are demonstrable in early childhood and continue to progress. Visual acuity is at its peak about age 20 and begins a decline about age 40. By age 50 almost everyone could benefit from some form of corrective lenses. Hearing also peaks about age 20 followed by a very gradual loss, usually at the high frequencies rather than the conversational levels. Some diminution in taste sense usually begins about age 50 and some loss of smell after age 40. Sensitivity to touch peaks about age 45 and then declines, but there is no accompanying loss of sensitivity to heat or cold.

These perceptual changes are well recognized, in general terms, when they are pronounced. However, the changes are usually subtle and therefore not necessarily recognized in one's self or in people with whom one is in daily contact. Since one of our goals as family physicians is to assist our patients in adapting and coping with changes in both the internal and external milieu, it is extremely important for us to be sensitive to such changes. Most difficulties in interactions appear to be related to faulty communication. When some of the basic tools for communication are damaged, it is important to recognize this and utilize compensatory mechanisms. It is also important to recognize that although changes in hearing and vision may be obvious to us, they may have been too gradual to be perceived by our patients or their family.

Sexual Perceptions

Understanding of changes in sexual behavior and attitudes during the course of adult development is essential. The impact of these changes is often exaggerated because of the importance of sexual activity as a

means of communication and self-perception, and of the current cultural emphasis on sexual activity. As family physicians we need most to know how to elicit sexual information and how to provide counseling, education, and sexual therapy to patients who wish it. More than specific information about sexual behavior, we need to be able to assess their meanings and the self-perceptions of patients and their partners.

A great wealth of information is available to physicians on sexual development. The changes frequently observed during female menopause are well known, including the great variations that are possible. The question of a male climacteric has never been fully agreed upon, but it is most important for us to recognize that in any individual a wide range of possibilities for change exist. It is also important for us to know, based on recent studies, that sexual activities usually continue throughout life, accompanied by sexually-related concerns. There is no point in life beyond which it would be inappropriate to elicit some form of sexual history concerning practices, concerns, and self-perceptions.

Intelligence

Intelligence includes many interrelated components, for which the measurement can be difficult. While approaches to measurement may be shown to have a high degree of validity for a given group, there is little assurance that such measurement will apply reliably to an individual. Nevertheless, some generalizations are of interest. Troll has pointed out that "at least some kinds of intellectual development may continue well past middle age. It is far from inevitable that we must get dumber as we get older. In fact, it is possible to get a lot wiser."[5] General intelligence testing provides an index of multiple skills and is referred to as omnibus testing. An example is the I.Q. obtained from a combination of scores on various subtests. Fluid intelligence could be considered the interaction between physiological ability and experience. This involves organizing and reorganizing information to solve problems. The growth curve would show a decline beginning at teenage. Crystalized intelligence results from the action of fluid intelligence on life experience and would be expected to increase throughout adulthood. Creativity, as another component of intelligence, shows great variation dependent on the kinds of creativity. Some creative activity, such as scientific research, is more dependent on crystalized rather than on fluid intelligence.

This is of great interest to those involved in studying the psychology of learning. As family physicians it is important only in realizing that great variation is possible among and within individuals. Attaching age-based labels can be blinding and destructive.

Available data indicates that the maintenance of memory function continues throughout the adult years.[5] Contrary to popular belief, there is little or no aging loss in long-term memory. Evidence is not so clear for short-term memory; there may be some loss in the amount of information that can be simultaneously stored for immediate access.

Complex mental problem-solving and reasoning, requiring the manipulation of information, may show some evidence of decline in late middle age. This may be balanced in older people by strategy. Thus, younger people may use less efficient problem-solving methods, such as trial and error. Older people, recognizing their slower processing, might first think the problem through; therefore, solve it with fewer false starts.

Coping

We have considered the biological changes of advancing age and the accompanying changes in learning, personality, and intellectual functioning. We have also considered the increasing health problems that accompany advancing age. Given the possibility of decreasing resources and increasing problems, how does the older person cope? What mechanisms are available and what opportunities are there for the health profession to assist?

Troll points out that coping can follow either of two general models. In some individuals it can be seen as a parallel curve to physical development reaching a highpoint in mid-years, then declining. This curve may be difficult to follow because of an opposite curve of increasing stress as years advance. This curve, and its downward arm, may gain momentum in individuals who continually cope poorly and seem to bring disaster on themselves. An alternate pattern is seen in individuals who learn early to cope with stress and whose ability to cope seems to grow based on each success. The curve is an upward curve as life advances and could continue as long as the individual has control of his or her major faculties.

In 1974, Maas and Kuypers published the results of a remarkable 40-year study. They followed the changes of 142 patients representing a variety of personality types and life styles all born about the turn of the century.[6] The basic findings of this study emphasize the distinctiveness and uniqueness of the individuals and of their methods of coping with life. Maas and Kuypers found no evidence of major decline in psychological functioning or of narrowing of life styles. Most of the patients are psychologically healthy and some have found increasing diversity of interests and experiences as their lives have increased. In summarizing their findings on both personality and life styles, as they correlate with health, they arrived at two conclusions: "First, health seems a crucial correlate of total personal functioning in old age. Second, early adult

health care may pay multiple dividends for old age—not only for health status then but also for aging personality dispositions and aging life styles."[6]

The first of these conclusions is not at all surprising, but the second reemphasizes the importance of helping patients understand, manage, and cope with their own health problems in early adult years, as well as the importance of providing optimum health care.

Social Attachments

Friends are chosen by adults more on the basis of life stage similarities than age. The friendships of adults have a tendency to persist over long periods of time even with interruptions in proximity. Best friends share intimate feelings, see each other frequently, and are likely to stay together over a long period of time.[5] Friendships serve as anchor points for adults within the larger society and provide a solid emotional support system. Troll quotes Loenthal and Haven (1968) that "old people who are able to maintain at least one intimate relationship can survive the drastic losses accompanying age that send the desolate friendless to the mental hospital."

Adults from middle age and onward are more likely to be involved in social organizations, partly because of freedom of time resulting from changed career activities and children leaving home. Increased involvement in social organizations may also be a reflection of increasing interest in societal activities, increasing awareness of one's own competence in contributing, and a sense of need for these organizations as a form of extended support system. In the author's experience these organizations—retirement clubs, hiking clubs, travel clubs, and study groups—form an extremely effective, major support system for many older adults.

The level of support which individuals seek from friends, society, and family presents another variable with great individual fluctuations. While there may be some cultural generalizations to be made (the concept of family has different implications in different ethnic groups), such generalizations are not likely to be helpful in understanding individual patients. Potential support systems and their meaning must be explored and understood on an individual basis.

Studies report a positive relationship overall between social engagement and life satisfaction.[7] Neugarten states:

It is our view that given a relatively supportive social environment, older persons like younger ones will choose the combinations of activities that offer them the most ego-involvement and are most consonant with their long established value patterns and self concepts. Aging is not a leveler of individual differences except, perhaps, at the very end of life. In adapting to both biological and social changes, the aging person continues to draw upon that which he has been as well as that which he is.

ROLE OF THE PHYSICIAN

As family health care providers, professionals trying to help people attain and maintain health, how can we be most helpful to our elderly patients? Brief consideration of some of the mechanisms and life attitudes of two patients who are coping extremely well may be helpful.

Mrs. Jessie L.*

Mrs. Jessie L. is a 95-year-old woman who has been a patient in my practice for 27 years. For the past 15 years she has been "head of the household" for a family including Ruth, a 40-year-old granddaughter with Down's Syndrome, and John, a 68-year-old son, with a variety of major health problems including alcoholism. The family subsists on a meager income. The major activities of the group consist of taking care of the home and the needs of each other. In spite of the obvious constraints, and occasional acute episodes of ill health with accompanying anxiety, the household is marked by pleasantry and an obvious sharing of affection for each other.

Jessie has made visits to the office every three to four months during the entire 27 years. Her general health has been excellent except for some of the perceptual problems of advanced age, musculoskeletal difficulties, and arteriosclerotic heart disease with various manifestations. Her mind is alert and lively and her sense of humor a joy to everyone. The staff enjoys her visits. Her occasional requests for home calls are usually soundly based.

Office visits are characterized by a sense of urgency: "Will I be alright for a while longer, Doctor? Ruth and John need me; I don't know what they would do without me." We have had numerous and detailed discussions on exactly what will be done when she dies. Her visits are usually brief, she has very few questions and follows advice to the best of her perception. Discussions usually include her current activities, a few basic health questions, and a series of questions about other members in the family. She professes no fear of dying, only regret for the suffering her departure will inflict on those who are dependent on her.

Dr. Alexander McDonald*

Dr. McDonald is a 97-year-old retired dentist who has been a mem-

* Names and some demographic data have been altered to assure confidentiality.

ber of the practice for 29 years. He has been active physically since a young man and continues a calisthenic routine on a daily basis. Mrs. McDonald is about 25 years younger than he but has been a semi-invalid for the past 12 years. Dr. McDonald retired from active practice in his late 70s, but did occasional consulting work for some years after that. He continues reading of dental journals and some professional activities. His principal current activities revolve around the care of his wife and their household.

Dr. McDonald's general health has been good although he also has moderate sensory loss and arteriosclerotic heart disease with various symptomatology. He visits the office regularly every three months. His visits are characterized by a series of questions concerning minor complaints, a discussion of his current and usually vigorous activities, and a lengthy discussion about his wife's current situation. He is a very religious man and our discussions often include an exchange of views on our spiritual beliefs.

Encounters with both individuals are characterized by a need for reassurance of their own health, not because of personal concern but because of concern over loved ones who are dependent on them. They both have an enormous and accurate sense of being needed. They are physically active in meeting these needs; both are keenly aware of their important roles; they are deeply involved in life with their families, friends, and neighbors. They have a highly developed sense of humor and seem much more focused on the present and future than on the past. Three kinds of coping mechanisms seem to be useful to them:

1. Social. There is a strong sense of purpose, of being absolutely necessary to others to whom they feel strongly attached. There is a palpable closeness with the family group and with a small group of friends. Within the close family group there is also freedom to "be one's self" without the overwhelming constraints of "don't do this" or "don't do that."
2. Spiritual. Older persons seem to have long ago come to terms in their relationships both to man and to God. This seems to be more than "making peace" but a real sense of joyful understanding and, to some degree, a joyful anticipation. Death is dreaded only in the sense that there is still much to be done for others here. Temporal troubles and tragedies can be met with the sure and certain confidence that they too are only temporary.
3. Emotional. There seems to be an ability to be aware of one's feelings, to share these feelings with others, and to tolerate differences in other people's perceptions.

As health coordinators we can learn much from our patients, particularly those who cope well. We can also support and reinforce the coping mechanisms that patients have developed or are trying to develop. Reinforcing such support may include actually being involved and allowing one's self to become a part of the patient's extended family.

REFERENCES

1. Vanderpool, JP: New visions of adulthood. Cont Ed 7:94–109, 1977
2. Sheehy G: *Passages*. New York: Dutton, 1976
3. Fried B: *The Middle-Age Crisis*. New York, Evanston and London: Harper & Row Publishers, 1967
4. Erikson E: "Eight Stages of Man." In *Childhood and Society*. New York: Norton, 1950
5. Troll, LE: *Early and Middle Adulthood*. Monterey: Brooks/Cole Publishing Company, 1975
6. Maas HS, Kuypers JA: *From Thirty to Seventy*. San Francisco: Jossey-Bass, Inc., Publishers, 1974
7. Neugarten BL: *Middle Age and Aging: A Reader in Social Psychology*. Chicago: The University of Chicago Press, 1968

CHAPTER 5

FAMILY DEVELOPMENT

JOHN P. GEYMAN AND JOE P. TUPIN

The book's second section will describe and discuss the development of individuals and families in order to lay the groundwork for consideration of diagnostic and management approaches to emotional and behavioral problems in family practice. The first two chapters dealt with the development of children and adults. This chapter addresses the development of the family as a dynamic and constantly changing entity with its own developmental features, quite different from those of individual family members.

Remarkable progress has been made by the medical specialty of pediatrics and the behavioral sciences during the past 30 years defining maturational stages of infants and children in terms of physical, emotional and behavioral development. Physicians have been better able to counsel patients and their families concerning normal development; thus recognizing and managing abnormal deviations and allaying fears stimulated by disruptive normal behavior. The development of adults and families has received considerably less attention, with most of the work in these areas confined to the sociologic and psychiatric literature.

Although the subject of family development is not yet well understood, it is possible to describe the basic emerging concepts that have clinical relevance to the family physician. The purpose of this chapter is threefold: (1) to present a concept of the family life cycle; (2) to describe the occurrence and impact of stress arising from predictable transitional crises; and (3) to summarize the implications of these concepts for the family physician.

FAMILY LIFE CYCLE

The concept of the family life cycle is based on several basic assumptions: (1) that families within our culture tend to have a beginning and an end; (2) that a number of distinct sequential phases can be recognized; and (3) that various phase-specific tasks can be delineated within each stage.[1] Within the family life cycle there is constant change of family members, interrelationships among family members, and the structure of the family itself.

The family life cycle represents the composite of individual developmental changes, evolution of the marital relationship, and development of the evolving family as a unit. Major events for an individual may create a crisis for the family, which is constantly reorganizing in response to multiple crises during each phase of family development. Examples include childbirth, adolescence, occupational change, major illness, disability, and death.

Crisis in this chapter refers to any event, personal or interpersonal, within or external to the family, requiring an adaptive response from the family unit. These events may be viewed as "good" or "bad" and may be transient or continuing. The family's response to such a crisis may be functional or dysfunctional. In their book, *Families In Crisis,* Glasser and Glasser note that those families which best respond to stress events usually exhibit three characteristics: (1) involvement (commitment to and active participation in family life by family members); (2) integration (interdependence of family members' roles); and (3) adaptation (flexibility and adaptive capabilities of the family's group structure and individual behaviors).[2]

Within the family life cycle, interesting observations have been made of marital and individual development. Rollins and Feldman studied levels of marital satisfaction over the family life cycle. They demonstrated similar highs and lows for wives and husbands, with troughs of lesser satisfaction during the mid-portion of the cycle[3] and higher levels of satisfaction early and late in the family life cycle. They found remarkably similar changes in individual satisfaction among wives and husbands at different stages of the family life cycle, again with similar lows during the mid-portion of the cycle.

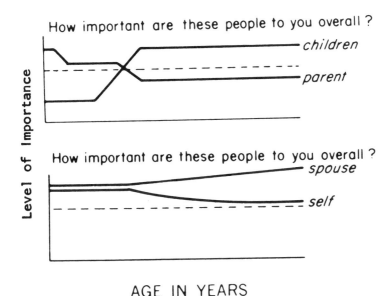

AGE IN YEARS

FIGURE 5-1. Sample curves associated with the time boundaries of the adult life span. (Adapted from Gould RL: The phases of adult life: A study of developmental psychology. Am J Psych 129:5, 1972.)

Recent studies of adult development have made important contributions to understanding some of the attitudinal and behavioral changes of aging adults. Gould's study of 524 healthy adults showed a number of rather striking changes between the ages of 20 and 60, all of which had direct and important effects on their families. Figure 5-1 illustrates sample curves for two selected parameters of adult attitudes over a 40-year period.[4]

In terms of duration of the various stages of the family life cycle, approximately one-half of the total life of the family is represented by the last two stages after the children are launched and the parents are left alone (Figure 5-2).[5, 6] These may be particularly critical stages in terms of stress and resultant clinical problems.

The family life cycle has been described in a number of ways. Table 5-1 shows five examples from the literature which vary from five to ten stages.

Although the classic nuclear family is used in this chapter to illustrate the principles of family development, these principles are likewise applicable to broader definitions of the family. Ransom and Vandervoort have defined the family as "a significant group of intimates, with a history and a future."[7] Smilkstein has defined the family as "adult partners, with

1. Newly Married
   (without children)
2. Birth of First Child
   (Oldest child, birth - 30 months)
3. Families with Preschool Children
   (Oldest child 30 months - 6 years)
4. Children in School
   (Oldest child 6 - 13 years)
5. Families with Teenagers
   (Oldest child 13 - 20 years)
6. Launching Years
   (First to last child leaving home)
7. Parents Alone
   (Last child gone - Retirement)
8. Retirement and Later Years
   (Retirement - Death of both spouses)

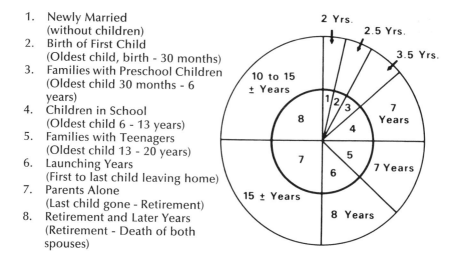

FIGURE 5-2.   The family life cycle by length of time in each of eight stages. (Adapted from Duvall EM: Family Development, 4th ed. Philadelphia, J. B. Lippincott Company, 151, 1971 as modified by Rakel RE: "The Family Life Cycle." In Principles of Family Medicine. Philadelphia, W. B. Saunders Company, 1977.)

or without children, and single parents with children—who have a sense of home and have an agreement to establish nurturing relationships."[8]

Regardless of the particular classification of the family life cycle which one finds most useful, they all have five basic developmental phases in common for every elementary family.

1. Birth of family. Elementary family originates with marriage of couple.
2. Phase of expansion. Begins with birth of first child and continues until the youngest child reaches adulthood. This phase includes the period of fertility, the period of physical and social maturation of children.
3. Phase of dispersion. Begins when the first child achieves adult status and continues until all children have grown and left home.
4. Phase of independence. Begins when all children have reached adulthood and left home so that the parents again live alone.
5. Phase of replacement. Begins when the parents retire from their major life roles and ends with their death. Usually includes a dependency stage of variable length.

Within each stage of the family life cycle, a number of predictable stage-specific tasks occur. As observed by Worby, "these tasks arouse

TABLE 5-1. Several Family Life Cycle Classifications*

Family Cycle Stage	National Conference on Family Life (1948)	Duvall (1957)	Rodgers (1962)	Worby (1971)	Solomon (1973)
1	Couple without children	Couple without children	Childless couple	Formation of Family	Marriage
2	Oldest child less than 30 months	Oldest child less than 30 months	All children less than 36 months	First child's birth	Birth of first child and subsequent child-bearing
3	Oldest child from 2½ to 5	Oldest child from 2½ to 6	Preschool family with (a) oldest 3–6 and youngest under 3, (b) all children 3–6	Early individuation of child	
4	Oldest child from 5 to 12	Oldest child from 6 to 13	School-age family with (a) infants, (b) preschoolers, (c) all children 6–13	Child's emerging sexuality	Individuation of family members
5	Oldest child from 13 to 19	Oldest child from 13 to 20	Teenage family with (a) infants, (b) preschoolers, (c) schoolagers, (d) all children 13–20	First child's adolescence	
6	When first child leaves till last is gone	When first child leaves till last is gone	Young adult family with (a) infants, (b) preschoolers, (c) schoolagers, (d) teenagers, (e) all children over 20		Actual departure of family

71

TABLE 5-1. Cont.

Family Cycle Stage	National Conference on Family Life (1948)	Duvall (1957)	Rodgers (1962)	Worby (1971)	Solomon (1973)
7	Later years	Empty nest to retirement	Launching family with (a) infants, (b) pre-schoolers, (c) school-agers, (d) teenagers, (e) youngest child over 20	Parents alone	Integration of loss
8			When all children have been launched until retirement		
9		Retirement to death of one or both spouses	Retirement until death of one spouse		
10			Death of first spouse to death of the survivor		

* Source: Rowe CP, The developmental conceptual framework to the study of the family. In Nye FI, Berardo IM: Emerging Conceptual Framework in Family Analysis. (New York: Macmillan, 1966) 208–209.

considerable stress within the family system and require of all family members a continuous mutual and reciprocal set of readjustments."[1] Table 5-2 outlines some of the important stage-specific tasks of the family life cycle described by Duvall.[5]

STRESS AND TRANSITIONAL CRISES

It is well recognized that the course of the family life cycle involves multiple stress points, particularly associated with major changes in the family unit and the transition from one stage to the next. Critical events such as divorce or death of a spouse precipitate crises within the family with resultant disequilibrium and need for reorganization. Previous roles and rules of intrafamily relationships frequently fail to maintain satisfactory family organization. New roles and rules must be established.

The process of family reorganization is often unpredictable and potentially disruptive. While the reorganized family may function as well as or better than before the crisis, the result of reorganization may be increased family dysfunction. Figure 5-3 graphically displays the response of a family to crisis resulting in a new level of family function.[9]

As a result of work with a social readjustment rating scale, Holmes has concluded that generalizations can be made about the relative stress on family life caused by various life crises. For example, of the normative crises, marriage, pregnancy and retirement are especially stressful. Divorce, separation, serious illness and death are the most stressful among nonnormative crises. Table 5-3 shows the relative stress ratings for various life events which have been derived from continued research over the years by Holmes and his colleagues.[10]

It should be noted that all of these crises are not necessarily or inherently "bad." Each of them, however, requires adaptation that causes intrafamily and individual adjustment, and this adaptation may be experienced by the participants as harmful. Individual variations in response to crises often reflect differing social and cultural values and individual psychological concerns and expectations. For example, the birth of a fourth child may create stress within the family if the mother came from a large family and the father came from a background where few children were the norm.

A generic classification of family crisis is shown in Table 5-4, which categorizes various kinds of crises within the family in terms of status shift, abandonment, addition and demoralization.[5, 11]

Depending on the outcome of the response of individual family members and the family as a whole, a given "normal" crisis may or may not cause a clinical problem perceived as requiring care by the individ-

TABLE 5-2. Stage-critical Family Developmental Tasks through the Family Life Cycle*

Stage of the Family Life Cycle	Positions in the Family	Stage-critical Family Developmental Tasks
1. Married couple	Wife Husband	Establishing a mutually satisfying marriage Adjusting to pregnancy and the promise of parenthood Fitting into the kin network
2. Childbearing	Wife-mother Husband-father Infant daughter or son or both	Having, adjusting to, and encouraging the development of infants Establishing a satisfying home for both parents and infant(s)
3. Preschool-age	Wife-mother Husband-father Daughter-sister Son-brother	Adapting to the critical needs and interests of preschool children in stimulating, growth-promoting ways Coping with energy depletion and lack of privacy as parents
4. School-age	Wife-mother Husband-father Daughter-sister Son-brother	Fitting into the community of school-age families in constructive ways Encouraging children's educational achievement
5. Teenage	Wife-mother Husband-father Daughter-sister Son-brother	Balancing freedom with responsibility as teenagers mature and emancipate themselves Establishing postparental interests and careers as growing parents

6. Launching center	Wife-mother-grandmother Husband-father-grandfather Daughter-sister-aunt Son-brother-uncle	Releasing young adults into work, military service, college, marriage, etc., with appropriate rituals and assistance Maintaining a supportive home base
7. Middle-aged parents	Wife-mother-grandmother Husband-father-grandfather	Rebuilding the marriage relationship Maintaining kin ties with older and younger generations
8. Aging family members	Widow/widower Wife-mother-grandmother Husband-father-grandfather	Coping with bereavement and living alone Closing the family home or adapting it to aging Adjusting to retirement

* Source: Duvall EM, Family Development, 4th ed. (Philadelphia: J. P. Lippincott Company, 1971)

76

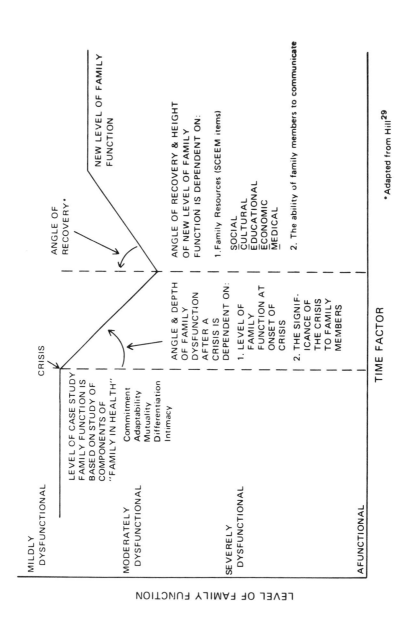

FIGURE 5-3. Schema for evaluation of family in crisis. (Adapted from Smilkstein G: The family in trouble: How to tell. J Fam Pract 2:1, 1975.)

TABLE 5-3. The Social Readjustment Rating Scale*

Life Event	Mean Value
1. Death of spouse	100
2. Divorce	73
3. Marital separation	65
4. Jail term	63
5. Death of close family member	63
6. Personal injury or illness	53
7. Marriage	50
8. Fired at work	47
9. Marital reconciliation	45
10. Retirement	45
11. Change in health of family member	44
12. Pregnancy	40
13. Sex difficulties	39
14. Gain of new family member	39
15. Business readjustment	39
16. Change in financial state	38
17. Death of close friend	37
18. Change to different line of work	36
19. Change in number of arguments with spouse	35
20. Mortgage over $10,000	31
21. Foreclosure of mortgage or loan	30
22. Change in responsibilities at work	29
23. Son or daughter leaving home	29
24. Trouble with in-laws	29
25. Outstanding personal achievement	28
26. Wife begin or stop work	26
27. Begin or end school	26
28. Change in living conditions	25
29. Revision of personal habits	24
30. Trouble with boss	23
31. Change in work hours or conditions	20
32. Change in residence	20
33. Change in schools	20
34. Change in recreation	19
35. Change in church activities	19
36. Change in social activities	18
37. Mortgage or loan less than $10,000	17
38. Change in sleeping habits	16
39. Change in number of family get-togethers	15
40. Change in eating habits	15
41. Vacation	13
42. Christmas	12
43. Minor violations of the law	11

* Source: Holmes TH, Rahe RH, The social readjustment rating scale. J Psychosom Res, 11:213–218, 1967

TABLE 5-4.   Generic Classification of Family Crisis*

Crises involving status shift	Sudden impoverishment Prolonged unemployment Sudden wealth or fame Political declassing
Crises of abandonment	Death of child or spouse Hospitalization of child or spouse Runaway Divorce
Crises of addition	Unwanted pregnancy Adoption Gain of stepfather, stepmother or stepsiblings Extended family or friends become household members
Crises of demoralization	Adultery Alcoholism Drug abuse Delinquency

*Source: Hill R: Generic features of families under stress. Soc Case 39:139–150, 1958 as modified by Smilkstein G: The family in trouble: How to tell. J Fam Pract 2:1, 1975

ual, family, or physician. Table 5-5 illustrates various kinds of clinical problems which can occur in response to critical events that are common in the course of a family's life cycle. This kind of conceptual framework can be useful to the family physician by increasing awareness of potential future crises in the individual patient and his/her family. It is well known that individuals with certain stress problems have a greater likelihood of developing other health problems as a result of future crises.

The family physician who knows patients and their families over a period of years has an excellent opportunity to anticipate, and prevent, stress illness in a family. Figure 5-4, for example, shows the relationship between the occurrence of paroxysmal atrial tachycardia to stress and other significant life events in one patient over a period of years.[12, 13]

IMPLICATIONS FOR THE FAMILY PHYSICIAN

It is widely accepted that family medicine is concerned with the comprehensive, ongoing care of individual patients and their families over the full course of the family life cycle. This deceptively simple goal is not attained in actual practice unless the family physician appreciates

TABLE 5-5.   Examples of Major Crises

Stage	"Normal" Crises	Clinical Problems
Birth of family	Early sexual adjustment	Sexual problems
Expansion of family		
Early (Preschool)	Birth of child	Postpartum depression
Middle (School)	Separation anxiety	Hyperactive child
Late (Adolescence)	Empty nest syndrome	Last fling
	Teenage identity crisis	Juvenile delinquency
Dispersion	Career stagnation	Depression
Independence	Menopause	Depression
	Marital readjustment	Alcoholism
	Death of parents	
Replacement	Physical disability	Organic brain syndrome
	Retirement	Depression
	Death of mate	Suicide
	Loneliness	

the family and its individual members as the patient. As Carmichael has observed: "to care for the patient in the context of the family is one thing; to turn the family into the object of care is another."[14]

This point is well illustrated by a common clinical example encountered daily in family practice. Many family physicians are skilled in recognizing depression in the individual patient and in individualizing the patient's management in the context of the family. It is quite another matter to pursue the next step toward diagnosis and management of related and possibly causative problems that exist within the family itself.

The family life cycle serves as a useful concept to understand and anticipate clinical problems within the family. Normal family development involves recurrent crises which are inevitable and predictable. It is important to appreciate that specific clinical problems, such as postpartum depression or post retirement depression, are correlated with particular stages of the family life cycle. It is also helpful to recognize that two or more stages of the family life cycle are often concurrent, as exemplified by a family with a depressed 45-year-old woman with empty nest syndrome, her 18-year-old son with an identity crisis, and her lonely, recently widowed 68-year-old mother.

Normal family development involves the completion of stage-specific tasks (Table 5-2) during each stage. Failure to complete these tasks

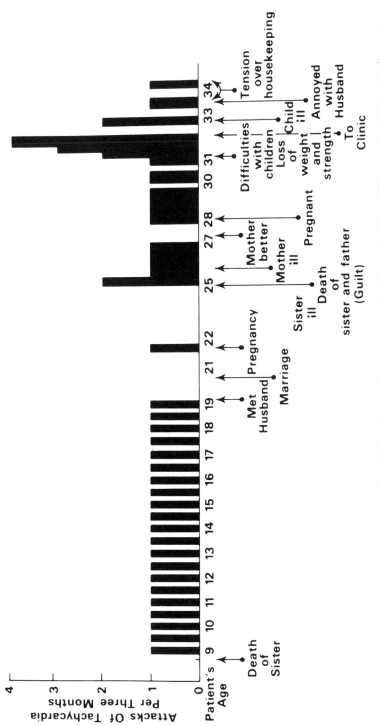

FIGURE 5-4. Relationships of paroxysmal atrial tachycardia to stress and other significant life events. (Adapted from Stevenson I: The Diagnostic Interview. 2nd Ed. New York, Harper and Row Publishers, 1971 as modified by Rakel RE: "Family Charting." In: Principles of Family Medicine. Philadelphia, W. B. Saunders Company, 1977.)

within a particular stage may lead to problems of adjustment within the next stages. Although multiple developmental stress points carry the potential for individual and family dysfunction, they may also lead to growth and improved levels of function within the family.

The family physician's clinical roles include preventive care, patient education, early diagnosis, medical management, and counseling on an individual and family basis. To provide this care, the family physician must integrate knowledge of the family and understanding of family dynamics with clinical knowledge and skills while perceiving the family, not the individual, as the patient.

REFERENCES

1. Worby CM: The family life cycle: An orienting concept for the family practice specialist. J Med Educ 46:3, 1971
2. Glasser PH and Glasser LN: *Families in Crisis*. New York: Harper and Row, 1971
3. Rollins BC, Feldman H: Marital satisfaction over the family life cycle. J Mar Fam 32:25, 1970
4. Gould RL: The phases of adult life: A study of developmental psychology. Am J Psych 129:5, 1972
5. Duvall, EM: *Family Development*. 4th ed. Philadelphia: J. B. Lippincott Company, 1971
6. Rakel RE: "The Family Life Cycle." In *Principles of Family Medicine*. Philadelphia: W. B. Saunders Company, 1977
7. Ransom DC and Vandervoort HE: The development of family medicine: Problematic trends. JAMA 225:1098, 1973
8. Smilkstein G: The family in trouble: How to tell. J Fam Prac 2:1, 1975
9. Geyman, JP: The family as the object of care in family practice. J Fam Prac 5:4, 1977
10. Holmes TH and Rahe RH: The social readjustment rating scale. J Psychosom Res 11:213, 1967
11. Hill R: Generic features of families under stress. Social Casework, 39:139, 1958
12. Stevenson I: *The Diagnostic Interview*. 2nd ed. New York: Harper and Row, 1971
13. Rakel RE: "Family Charting." In *Principles of Family Medicine*. Philadelphia: W. B. Saunders Company, 1972
14. Carmichael LP: The family in medicine, process or entity? J Fam Pract 3:562, 1976

CHAPTER 6

CLINICAL APPLICATIONS OF A DEVELOPMENTAL FRAMEWORK

CHARLES KENT SMITH, JACK MARTIN REITER,
AND BURTON V. REIFLER

This chapter applies a developmental framework to the clinical work of the family physician, using the work of Erik H. Erikson.[1] Erikson's eight stages of personality development present human growth within a framework that permits presentation of clinical examples of development. In this model the development of the personality unfolds in phases, though not at a steady pace. The person goes through periods of relative quiet and then marked change as he or she moves into a new phase of life, opening new potentials, new areas to explore, new challenges to master, and requiring new sets of skills and abilities. There is a repetitive pattern in how the same individual is likely to surmount various crises later in life.

At each stage the person faces in two directions with opposing motivations, and with each stage failure to cope with the essential tasks of that phase leaves the person unprepared to move forward. Most commonly a person moves ahead in some spheres but makes repetitive efforts to master tasks from the earlier stages.

STAGE ONE: TRUST VERSUS BASIC MISTRUST

A critical task and central theme of infancy concerns the establishment of feelings of confidence in the world. The child needs to gain a sense that those upon whom it unknowingly depends are dependable. Either a basic trust in others is attained, which forms the basis for achieving trust in self, or an enduring distrust may develop. If essential needs are met, the child gains a feeling that the world is trustworthy and adequately consistent.

Children who are indulged as infants may acquire a lasting and inappropriate optimism that prevents them from providing for themselves, since they feel certain that others will look out for them. Those who have been deprived and frustrated may have a deep-seated pessimism, becoming hostile and resentful when their needs are not met.

STAGE TWO: AUTONOMY VERSUS DOUBT AND SHAME

This stage lasts approximately 18 months through 3 years. Emphasis in the second year of life is on the attainment of muscular control in general. In learning self-control the child properly gains a lasting sense of autonomy, or loses self-esteem and develops a pervasive sense of doubt and shame.

As the baby emerges from infancy and starts to walk and talk, a new phase is entered in which crucial problems develop from an imbalance between new found motor skills and meager mental capacities. Limits must be placed upon activities for the child's safety and for the preservation of family possessions. The relationship with the mother changes accordingly. During infancy she has nurtured the child, provided for its needs, and encouraged its wanderings; she must now set limits.

A mother who finds her child's activities anxiety provoking may overly limit the child, surrounding it with a barrier of "no's" that stifle initiative and self-confidence. Mothers who lack confidence in their ability to guide and control the child are apt to project such feelings and magnify the child's incapacity to care for itself. Mothers who cannot tolerate disorder, or overestimate the baby's capacity to conform and regulate impulses, can convey a sense of "being bad" to the child; and provoke a sense of guilt and shame that undermines feelings of worth and self-trust. The child may be led into an over-conformity that satisfies the parents but covers hostile resistance and stubbornness.

At the end of this period, a relatively good equilibrium has been established between the child's motor and linguistic abilities. The child is ready to gain a more definitive autonomy from its mother and find a place as a member of the family.

STAGE THREE: INITIATIVE VERSUS GUILT

Erikson considers the basic issues of the third period to involve the balance between initiative and guilt, initiative being concerned with becoming a person through identification with the father or mother, guilt deriving largely from rivalry with the father and siblings for the mother. Greater independence brings greater insecurity in its wake. Thumb sucking is more common at 4 than at 2 or 3, and there are other behaviors indicating regression toward babyish ways and former security. Concerns over death may occur; this is an extension of "separation anxiety." Dreams and reality are not separable and many children now seek the comfort and safety of the parents' bed in the middle of the night. These concerns heighten as the child approaches 5.

The resolution of this period terminates early childhood. The child has taken a giant step toward becoming an independent and self-sufficient person. There is a consolidation of the child's personality as some integration as an individual is achieved. To function effectively outside of the family, the child must have become capable of delaying gratification and must also have learned the essentials of socialization.

STAGE FOUR: INDUSTRY VERSUS INFERIORITY

During school years where gaining admiration, approval, and affection depends upon achievement, the child must acquire a sense of industry or become subject to a sense of inferiority. This stage is enclosed by the danger of habitual compulsive striving to excel, by defeatist trends, and an unwillingness to accept and face meaningful challenges. Other character traits also appear to have their roots in this period of life. The child acquires a sense of belonging and the assurance of acceptance as part of the group, and of the larger society, in contrast to feeling like an outsider. A sense of responsibility also develops at this stage, with the willingness and capacity to live up to the expectations of others. The child has become sufficiently independent to be on its own, exploring new interests, and moving into real or imaginary ventures assuming few responsibilities. The child is being weaned from home, and learning to feel comfortable and secure while interdependent with others.

The school has the function of teaching the child the knowledge and skills required in order to function as a reasonably self-sufficient adult in society. It is a major socializing agency, taking over from the family and implementing its functions. The school serves as the first significant institution which differentiates children on the basis of achievement; the parents theoretically have accepted the child simply because it is theirs, an acceptance and affection which the child continues to need in order to feel emotionally secure. The school introduces different and more impartial standards than the home, and also presents community values. The danger at this stage lies in a sense of inadequacy and inferiority. This period ends with a new spurt and physical growth that precedes the onset of puberty when the child begins to become an adolescent.

STAGE FIVE: IDENTITY VERSUS ROLE DIFFUSION

It is difficult to convey what transpires during the years of adolescence, in which the child blossoms into an adult beset by conflicting emotions, struggling to maintain self-control and achieve self-expression, under the impact of sensations and impulses that are scarcely understood. It is a time of seeking, seeking inward to find who one is, searching outward to locate one's place in life, and longing for others with whom to satisfy cravings for intimacy and fulfillment.

Unfortunately, there is a tendency to overread adolescence as a period of extreme psychopathology. At the start of adolescence the child is still at play, dependently attached to the family, and has an undefined future. At the end of adolescence, the child has developed responsibility for self, a personality pattern has been established, and life goals may be taking shape.

One of Erikson's major contributions to developmental psychology was his emphasis upon the importance of late adolescence. The young person must now obtain an identity in his or her own right, not simply as someone's son or daughter. This period involves considerable trying out, and an implicit understanding that one is not yet playing for keeps. Failure in adolescence leads to role diffusion and an inability to settle on an occupational identity.

STAGE SIX: INTIMACY AND ISOLATION

Erikson's sixth formal stage corresponds with the expansion phase outlined in Chapter 6. If a person's identity is secure, he or she will be capable of involvement with others in meaningful ways without the threat of losing his or her own sense of identity. In this regard, marriage and childbirth test the successful passage through earlier stages.

STAGE SEVEN: GENERATIVITY VERSUS STAGNATION

This stage deals in the broadest sense with the person's interest in making a contribution to society.

STAGE EIGHT: INTEGRATION VERSUS DESPAIR

In the eighth stage, the stage of maturity, a person assesses the way he or she has lived and contributed to society. Integration/integrity will be prominent if a person feels that past years have been lived productively and responsibly. Despair results if dissatisfaction exists with life's accomplishments.

CASE ILLUSTRATIONS

It is clear from the above summary of Erikson's stages of life that the environment, temperament, genetic givens, and other as yet undefined factors all play a role in an individual's growth and development. The following case studies are examples of patients' strengths and weaknesses that are due to the above factors.

Bill S

Bill is a 15-year-old boy. His parents both work, and have generally been seen for only acute illnesses. Mrs. S has had three visits over the past month for headaches and Dr. A considers them tension headaches. His general inquiry about the family elicits a flood of information about Bill.

Mrs. S was distraught. Bill had been truant from school twice, became intoxicated on several weekends, and has grown more reclusive and secretive. His parents suspect that he uses drugs.

The two older children did not experience similar problems. Their adolescent rebellion had been stormy, but involved more shouting than acting out. Mrs. S did not know what to do about Bill, and felt she was failing as a mother. Mr. S was considering corporal punishment.

Dr. A sought more information from his files, augmented by information from Mrs. S. Bill had appeared to gain a sense of basic trust, and at the appropriate age he had mastered control of toilet training and other motor functions. A sense of initiative had been apparent from his parents' reports of his early play. A few problems cropped up during his initial school years. These were largely resolved as Bill was given adequate attention by his teachers and became respected for his industriousness.

Dr. A wondered if Bill's behavior might be part of the next stage of development: identity versus role diffusion. Mrs. S responded by commenting that she never knew what Bill would do next; first it was guitar, then football, then old cars. Deciding to assume that Bill was going through a normative developmental stage, Dr. A elected to defer any consideration of psychiatric disorder until following the family over a longer period. He reassured Mrs. S that she was acting as a good parent and offered to talk to Bill, if he would come to the office.

Bill's initial appearance was disappointing, going beyond the adolescent uniform of careful sloppiness. Dr. A questioned the initial assumptions he had held when meeting with Mrs. S but a 30-minute conversation proved very revealing. Bill had formed an intense loyalty to an older boy, Dave, who had dropped out of school. He felt that Dave was tough and cool and knew how to get what he wanted.

Dr. A listened carefully and asked about Dave's future, and whether Bill saw himself being Dave's follower a year from now. Dr. A believed that Bill's attachment to Dave would not last, but that serious trouble could arise before it ended. He related this in a straightforward manner: "Bill, I know you feel you have a good friend, but stay alert and keep your head. I can't tell you not to use drugs because if your mind is made up you won't listen. However, I have seen other boys in your situation go in two different directions. Some ride it out unharmed; others get in over their heads. I suggest you stay open-minded and keep your choices open by sticking with your sports and getting your car ready for when you get your driver's license. If you eventually decide that Dave's life style is for you, then that's your business."

The next six months were difficult for all parties involved. Bill continued to defy his parents' authority, but seemed to hold off on drinking and made it to school every day. Eventually, he moved on to other, healthier pursuits. While his grades had suffered temporarily, he had averted more serious difficulties.

Mr. and Mrs. Jones

Mr. and Mrs. Jones had been married for five years. The marriage was stable and both were working in a local aircraft factory. Their daughter was born after a normal pregnancy. At delivery, the child was noted to have a cleft palate and some associated abnormalities that made feeding and swallowing difficult. The mother pumped her breasts initially, but after a short time switched to a high calorie formula. Feeding continued to be a significant problem and there was a constant threat of aspiration. Feeding by gavage was considered, but rejected by the mother for a variety of reasons, predominantly having to do with bonding with the infant. Medically, the course proved to be stable. At approximately 1 year, recurrent otitis media necessitated bilateral myringotomy with insertion of tubes. This was performed uneventfully. At two years a palatal repair was undertaken with complete success. Her growth and development proceded normally, although speech may have been slightly behind normal developmental parameters.

It appeared to Dr. P that there was a significant potential for interference with adequate bonding of mother and daughter. Dr. P was also concerned about overprotectiveness as a way of dealing with the child's disability. He thought it desirable to work closely with both parents to establish a basic trust between the infant and parents, and to aid the child's later development of a sense of autonomy. Thus, it was important that the child was loved despite physical abnormalities, but not overloved to stifle her self-confidence. The family worked with the doctor, nurse, and social worker and responded very positively.

During the myringotomy and the palate repair professional support was given. After the surgeries, close contact with the family was maintained so the girl would not be handicapped as she moved toward development of autonomy and intiative (Stage 3). Finally, the parents were supported and the child seen regularly as her need to belong to a peer group increased. The Eriksonian stages were reviewed with the parents and this proved helpful in assuring the child's normal development.

John S

John was born while both parents were experiencing extreme emotional illness and constant bickering. When John first came for counseling, he could only speak about his father's drinking problem and his parents' continual battling. John appeared to have moderate intellectual impairment and was extremely inhibited for a 10-year-old boy. Psychological testing placed his I.Q. at the lower end of the mildly retarded range.

Counseling was conducted to assist with John's adjustment. In many respects, John had a firmer grip on reality than did his parents. Accordingly, the first half of each session was spent discussing the previous week's home occurrences. Alternative ways to act and understand these events were discussed during the second half of the session. By having someone listen to him for the first time in his life, John was able to blossom in many areas of his functioning. At the same time, this became a threat to his parents.

Progress with the family was very slow but continued to have an upward slope. Mr. S was begun on Amitriptyline and, within two to three weeks, had an excellent response with marked decrease in drinking. Based on historical information, it appeared possible that Mrs. S's disorder was of the manic-depressive type. Lithium carbonate was used with dramatic reversal of the dysfunctional signs and symptoms. Stabilizing both parents' emotional status allowed for a dramatic change in the family. Both parents advanced in their careers. John began to test out his environment in more normal, and occasionally exaggerated, adolescent ways. Psychological testing was repeated and John's I.Q. score was no longer in the dull normal range. It was clear that the earlier results were to a large part influenced by the intellectual deprivation that John had received at home. With the provision of twice weekly tutoring, John's horizons are expanding considerably.

The A Family

To further illustrate the process of human development and the interpersonal factors that influence and modify it, the following example involves three generations: the elderly grandparents, their middle-aged children, and their adolescent grandchildren. The possible permutations for adaptations to the tasks proposed by Erikson are legion within a given family; therefore the peculiarities of this example serve only as an introduction to the developmental process. This is a case of the intellectual decline of an older person. How each member of the family views this event and how it affects relationships within the family, is complex.

The situation's complexity becomes more manageable if individual reactions are understood within the context of the adaptational tasks faced by each member of the family.

Mr. and Mrs. A were each 75 years of age. During Mr. A's fifties and sixties his needs for accumulation of money and influence had gradually given way to interest in his family and community. Earlier, Mr. A had worried about matters like financing college educations and his value as an employee. He had also tried to come to grips with his own mortality, a dilemma particularly heightened by the death of his own parents. As time passed, his priorities shifted, his interests constricted somewhat, and he became more accepting and less preoccupied with the reality of his lifespan.

At 70, Mr. A retired. Dr. M, his physician over the past 20 years, pronounced his general health as excellent. He advised him not to make any permanent geographic moves for at least one year, and to take one major change at a time. When Mr. A commented to Dr. M that he was being put to pasture, Dr. M responded supportively that this need not be the case, and then asked Mr. A if this was really how he felt. As Dr. M had guessed, Mr. A was ambivalent, experiencing the loss of his working identity, but also feeling a sense of integrity that had been developing over his senior adult years. Through briefly ventilating this ambivalence, the healthy aspect of this adaptational task emerged.

At age 74, the situation changed. Mr. A's memory began to fail, he would get lost on short walks, and he began to suspect his family and neighbors of stealing his possessions. His family tried to cope with the situation, despite their lack of knowledge about cognitive impairment.[2] They felt very strongly about doing everything they could to avoid institutionalization.[3]

Dr. M was consulted, and began his evaluation with a thorough history and physical examination appropriate to cognitive impairment. He inquired about transient neurologic deficits that might suggest tumor or hydrocephalus, asked about medications that could lead to intoxication, and sought information about episodes of depression, which in the elderly can masquerade as dementia. Physical examination and laboratory tests ruled out deficiency states, endocrine disorders, infections, and neurological disease. The diagnosis of exclusion was therefore senile dementia.

Responses from the family varied. Through Dr. M's knowledge of the natural history of the illness, the personalities of the family members, and the adaptational tasks each member faced, Dr. M was able to assist the family in coping; thereby preserving as much of Mr. A's function as possible and keeping him at home.

Mrs. A responded with resolution and determination. After a lifetime of companionship, loneliness was her greatest concern. While she recognized that she would likely outlive her husband, she still wanted to invest as much energy in the relationship as possible. Dr. M felt that her dedication was crucial and elected to assist rather than suggest the task was too great. Among his suggestions were teaching Mr. A landmarks for turning on his walks, and providing a guide rope from the bed to the bathroom to avoid middle of the night disorientation.

Dr. M was more concerned about the younger generations in the family. Mr. A's son was initially hostile to Dr. M, suggesting that further tests would surely reveal the cause of his father's decline. Dr. M suspected that the son was actually worried about the impact of his father's illness on his own future; both the financial burden he would have to bear, and if the problem were hereditary. Mr. A's son was at a stage where preparation for the future generations was crucial, and his power to accomplish this was now threatened by his father's illness. Dr. M managed this through practical advice about lack of certainty concerning familial tendencies in cognitive impairment, and through realistically addressing the son's concerns.

Mr. A's daughter-in-law had developed a new career over the previous five years as her children became enrolled in school full time. She wished to continue this, but felt guilty about not helping more with Mr. A. Dr. M was able to address this by reassuring her that Mr. and Mrs. A were managing well generally, and were getting assistance from a variety of community services. He commented that her continuing to see them socially at the same frequency as before was all that was needed for the present.

The 17-year-old grandson was confused. His image of his grandfather was one of strength and kindness. As his grandfather declined, he began to argue more vehemently with his parents over trivial matters. This seemed to be out of character for him and his mother mentioned it to Dr. M. At a later office visit by the grandson for a minor problem, Dr. M brought up the subject of his grandfather, and the reason for the outbursts became clearer. The grandson now saw Mr. A as weak and powerless and blamed his father for letting it happen. As he wished his own identity to be strong and resourceful, the reality of his grandfather's decline and his father's powerlessness to halt it induced fear and resentment. Dr. M pointed out that truly resourceful people channel their frustration into constructive outlets. He suggested the grandson face the problem directly by returning the kindness his grandfather had shown him. The grandson was reluctant, but made an effort to do as suggested with eventual good results.

Had Dr. M not provided for each family member a measure of support, the family cohesiveness and care provided to Mr. A might have suffered needlessly. Since Dr. M anticipated that each family member would view the situation from an individual perspective, he reasoned that an individual approach was required. This approach involved no direct psychotherapy in the sense of regularly scheduled counseling sessions. Rather, it took the form of reallocation of office visit time. Since Dr. M anticipated many of the concerns family members had, he was able to address them quickly and effectively. He pointed out that each relative had a particular point of view, and was able to encourage communication and mutual support.

CONCLUSION

Family physicians relate simultaneously with patients ranging in age from infancy to old age, who in turn are dealing with members of their own families. In order to grasp character and personality growth shaped within the chrysalis of family and society, the family physicians must be aware of the many ways of dealing with human development from the classical Freudian approach to the more behavioral and learning models.[4, 5, 6] These models are certainly not exclusive of each other and they have been summarized elsewhere.[7]

The Eriksonian framework is one approach that seems uniquely suitable for use by family physicians. It can be easily understood and shared with parents and their families and covers the entire life cycle. It is family oriented and realizes the impact of societal factors as well.

The case illustrations presented in this chapter demonstrate the practical value of such a framework. The physician can understand and use this framework to help families cope with a wide variety of difficulties.

REFERENCES

1. Erikson EH: *Childhood and Society.* 1st ed. New York: W. W. Norton & Co., 1963
2. Williams TF, Hill JH, Fairbank MD, Know KG: Appropriate placement of the chronically ill and aged. JAMA, 226:1332, 1973
3. Issacs B: Geriatric patients: Do their families care? British Med Jour 4:282, 1971
4. Freedman A, Kaplan H: *Comprehensive Textbook of Psychiatry.* 2nd ed. Baltimore: Williams and Williams, 1976
5. Vaillant GE: *Adaptation to Life.* Boston: Little, Brown, 1977
6. Sheehy G: *Passages.* New York: Dutton, 1976
7. Lidz T: *The Person.* New York: Basic Books, Inc., 1976

SECTION III

Approaches to Diagnosis

CHAPTER 7

PSYCHOSOCIAL ISSUES IN ASSESSMENT

ARTHUR KLEINMAN AND GABRIEL SMILKSTEIN

The aim of this chapter is to outline psychosocial issues that need to be assessed routinely in family medicine and primary care; to construct what we consider a practicable framework with which clinicians can conceptualize, investigate, and respond to applicable problems.

Psychosocial diagnosis should encompass the behavioral status of an individual, family structure and function, ethnicity, social status, role relationships, and coping response to sickness and other stress. The behavioral status of the individual is extensively covered in the psychiatric literature [1-3] and has received adequate treatment in family medicine.[4-6] The diagnosis of individual behavioral status includes an assessment of mental status in terms of personality type, affective state, language, memory and cognition, behavioral style and performance. It also includes such specific psychopathological features as delusions, hallucinations, phobias, reality testing and suicidal status. This assessment also attempts to rule out such common psychiatric problems as the depressive syndrome; hysteria and other forms of somatization; acute and chronic psychotic conditions (e.g., schizophrenia and manic-depressive psychosis); organic brain syndromes; sexual deviances; and related conditions.[7, 8] When a behavioral aberration is present, clinical investigation is needed to see if it is a primary psychological problem (e.g., hysteria) or a problem secondary to organic disorders (e.g., depression as a presenting complaint in diabetes, personality disorder and schizophrenia in temporal lobe epilepsy, or catatonia in a metabolic encephalopathy).[9] As in the treatment of medical disorders, the treatment of psychosocial problems requires the clinician to formulate an assessment and begin a treatment plan.

Assessment of family structure and function is covered in Chapter 10 and will not be discussed here. Within a unified psychosocial framework, we shall examine how the clinician can evaluate and manage problems relating to patients' ethnicity, social status, role, interpersonal relationships, and coping response to sickness and other life stresses. In this manner, we respond to Engle's charge that medical care requires a new and broader model aware of social and cultural interrelationships as well as biological and psychological variables.[9, 10]

The framework is based upon research carried out by medical anthropologists, medical sociologists, social psychologists, and other medical social scientists.[11–13] It also represents the effort of clinicians (some of whom are also behavioral scientists) to translate social science concepts and strategies into usable clinical categories and treatment interventions.[11, 14, 15]

DISEASE PROBLEMS AND ILLNESS PROBLEMS

A fundamental distinction exists between the disease and illness aspects of sickness. Disease means the biological abnormality underlying sickness; illness means the way the patient (and members of his family and social network) perceives, labels, experiences, evaluates, and responds to symptoms. From this perspective, illness is always specific to a particular individual in a particular family, social class, and ethnic niche. Social structure and cultural norms mainly affect sickness and patient care by influencing how patients experience and react to sickness and treatment plans. The response of patients and families to illness affects epidemiological patterns of disease, because it shapes the presentation of symptoms, their course, and the outcome of illness.

Disease problems are what most clinicians routinely note in patient charts as the signs or causes of sickness. For example, they include status of blood sugar and required insulin dosage in patients with diabetes, reports of skin test results and respiratory tests in asthmatic patients, side-effects of various prescribed medications, and reasons for and results of biological tests or surgical procedures.

Illness problems, on the other hand, may or may not be routinely

recorded in the problem-oriented record. They might include the following:

1. Maladaptive coping responses patients and families use to manage
    sickness, such as denial, passive-hostile behavior, "shopping" among
    different doctors, and suicidal attempts.[16]
2. Financial problems created or worsened by sickness.
3. Family problems created or worsened by sickness.
4. Major social role changes in a person experiencing a terminal sick-
    ness or a permanent disability.
5. Inappropriate resort to sick role and illness behavior due to psycho-
    logical or social gain.
6. Conflict in personal beliefs between patients, family, and practi-
    tioners concerning course or nature of sickness and objectives for
    treatment.
7. Conflict in cultural values concerning treatment style and interper-
    sonal etiquette between ethnic patients and practitioners due to
    substantial differences in social class and life style.
8. Lack of compliance with therapeutic regimen due to the unusual
    nature of a procedure or its expected outcome.
9. Inappropriate use of alternative or indigenous health care agents
    and agencies.
10. Breakdown in communication between patient, family, and practi-
    tioner.
11. Transference and counter-transference problems in the doctor-
    patient or doctor-family relationship.
12. Special life problems stemming from stresses engendered by the
    environment.

Although illness problems are almost as varied as disease problems,
the examples described represent the major categories. By systematically
assessing illness problems and recording them in the problem-oriented
record, physicians not only will evaluate how patient and family cope
with sickness and respond to clinical care; they will be able to target
interventions more specifically, as we shall describe below. Integrated
comprehensive care should mean that both disease and illness problems
are elicited, treated, and evaluated at follow-up.

ASSESSMENT OF ILLNESS PROBLEMS

Illness problems can be routinely assessed in the following way:

1. The coping responses of the patient and family to illness should
be examined.[16, 17] Part of this examination should include assessment of
habitual coping responses to previous stress, including previous sickness.

Special attention should be directed to maladaptive coping mechanisms used by the sick person and family. Coping responses involve (i) cognitive processes, sometimes called ego defenses, such as denial, somatization and other forms of displacement, projection, dissociation, and reaction formation; (ii) positive behavioral responses (e.g., search for and utilization of available information, active participation in self-care, use of relevant social agencies); and (iii) negative behavioral responses (e.g., acting out, passive-hostile behavior, noncompliance).

   2.   The clinician should assess both the childhood and adult developmental period the patient is in and the impact of illness and treatment on the chief developmental issues of that period (e.g., autonomy and formation of personal identity in late adolescence).[18, 19]

   3.   Illness problems relating to the family life cycle have been identified as an area of interest and study central to family medicine.[20, 21] A problem such as diabetes will manifest a different set of disease-illness concerns according to the time in the life cycle[1] it is evaluated and treated. For example, the diabetes disease concerns of an adolescent will probably relate to fluctuating blood sugar level, while the illness problems may relate to compliance issues associated with adolescent rebellion. The disease-illness variations in diabetes may be so great through the life cycle, one may wonder if it is the same sickness.

   4.   The clinician needs to elicit patient and family explanations for the given illness episode, the beliefs and expectations they hold about cause, onset, pathophysiology, and course of the disorder. This is of particular importance when treating patients from distinctive ethnic and social class backgrounds whose illness beliefs and values frequently differ from biomedical ones. These issues can be elicited by direct questioning (see questions formulated by Kleinman, Eisenberg, and Good).[14] Discrepancies and conflicts can be brought to the surface if the physician demonstrates warmth, empathy, and a genuine interest in hearing the patient's perspective. Negotiating is frequently required to achieve a compromise between patient and practitioner viewpoints. Since medicine is itself a "culture" with its own system of norms and meanings that may conflict with the popular point of view, it is worth the physician's time to elicit the patient's explanation of the illness episode by asking what they think is wrong and why.

   Related to this, the physician should elicit patient and family treatment objectives, which may diverge from those of the physician. Again, negotiation is essential to work out a feasible treatment plan that is rational, potentially effective, and likely to be followed. Although there are no specific rules for conducting such a therapeutic negotiation, experience is that establishing this as the ethos of care is a major step in diminishing patient-doctor miscommunication and tacit conflicts leading to noncompliance and patient dissatisfaction.

It needs re-emphasizing that both patient and family explanations should be elicited. Often the physician may find discrepancies or conflict. The result can be major management problems adversely affecting the course of sickness and treatment plan. In this instance, the physician should mediate between patient and family point of view as part of therapeutic negotiation.

5.   The clinician should evaluate the significance of the illness for the patient and family. It is useful to apply the model developed by Lipowski that illness can have any of four meanings for patients.[17] These meanings include such combinations as no major significance, threat, loss, and gain. The first three can be assessed through direct questioning. The last usually requires additional observation and information regarding the patient's usual role and the changes induced by illness.

6.   Another important stage in assessment is of concern to those clinicians who routinely see patients from given ethnic groups. This physician needs to become aware of the ethnic group's key illness beliefs, treatment expectations, and rules governing communicative etiquette and interpersonal transactions. Much of this material is available in the medical anthropological literature,[22-24] and some has been written in papers that can be used directly.[25]

7.   The clinician should remove common structural barriers in patient-doctor communication. This means a number of things. The medical explanation must be translated into language the patient can understand, and there must be ample time allotted for patients to assimilate the material and raise questions. The value of this procedure has been validated in compliance studies.[26] Part of the problem in clinical communication is overcome when the physician accepts the doctor-patient interaction as a two-way communication involving biomedical and popular languages of medicine that potentially distort messages and require translation as well as repetition. The countervailing biomedical view of the doctor as a learned expert and the client as a passive recipient of knowledge has been a persistent source of mischief in clinical communication.

The physician can facilitate communication further by establishing a permissive atmosphere that allows patients to reveal ideas and values they feel might cause ridicule or intimidation.

Given the frequency of communicative problems in health care, the physician is at an advantage to anticipate them. Data show that two major variables improve patient compliance. One variable is high informational content provided by the physician. The other is the ongoing motivation of patients to comply as a consequence of the physician's anticipating and monitoring noncompliance.[26-28]

8.   The physician should recognize that family function can worsen, remain unchanged, or even improve, under the stress of sickness. He should be prepared to diagnose and manage family problems, or where

appropriate, refer patients to experts and treatment agencies (see Chapter 10). Similarly, recognition of a resource-poor family should be followed by adjustment of the treatment plan and referral to appropriate community agencies. Families with a poverty of resources can be overwhelming management problems, but the physician's responsibility is to recognize the problems and suggest resources that can offer assistance.

9. When illness results in major changes from pre-morbid social status and role, or when the sick role is used inappropriately by patient or family to sanction such change (e.g., failure in business or school), the physician can work out suitable plans to help patients avoid maladaptive coping strategies (e.g., somatization producing chronic learned pain in a depressed patient with a marital problem).[9] For many patients chronic sickness means loss of self-esteem, major change in identity or body image, or an impaired state preventing normal role performance at work and in the family. Treatment may require the physician to give more attention to the psychosocial management of these key illness problems, as well as the use of a biomedical approach to treat the underlying disease. Balint has argued that these illness problems require the use of the physician's own personality as a therapeutic device. He suggests the establishment of a therapeutic alliance accompanied by supportive psychotherapy and perhaps behavior modification techniques.[29]

10. Frequently, the physician is enmeshed in very difficult family and social network entanglements between patients and bureaucratic institutions. These may be conceptualized best and perhaps resolved by comparing how the physician and patient label sickness. These problems are illustrated in Table 7-1. Situations represented by quadrants I and IV usually present no problems to primary care givers. Patient, family, and care giver agree on the same label—the patient is sick or well. The conflict situations represented by quadrants II and III, however, can be major problems in primary care. Here either the physician, or some other

TABLE 7-1. Patterns of Sickness Labels*

Label applied by family, physician, or social agencies	Label Applied by Patient	
	Sick	Well
Sick	I	II
Well	III	IV

* Modified from Twaddle[30]

labeler, and the patient are in basic disagreement over whether the patient is sick or well. Since these conflicts are usually worsened by the anxieties or insecurities of both patient and physician, as well as family members and institutions, it is important that the primary care physician avoid entering an adversary relationship by "taking sides." Recognizing discrepancies is the first and perhaps most important step in resolving them.

Medical euphemisms and pejorative expressions such as denial, chronic functional complaints, and "crock," obscure the fact that the conflicts described are problems in social transactions determining whether or not the patient will be given the rights and responsibilities of the sick role. Proper management of such problems flows from the physician's willingness to investigate as legitimate, even if he disagrees, various points of view on labeling sickness.

11.   Recognition of discrepancies in patient and practitioner evaluations of therapeutic outcomes is another important task for the primary care physician. Several studies have shown that when patient and doctor disagree as to what constitutes effective care, a negative outcome may result.[31, 32] The primary care physician should routinely assess such conflicts between professional and lay medical cultures. When present, these conflicts should be negotiated. Thus, the doctor may have employed purely technical biological criteria to establish if treatment was effective; the patient interpreted outcome in terms of improvement in the psychosocial burden of disease. Assessment of potentially discrepant views of therapeutic outcome is particularly desirable when patient and doctor do not share the same culture, social class, or life-style.

12.   An important illness problem area involves self-care and health maintenance. Studies reveal that 70 to 90 percent of all illness episodes are managed by the family and social network without recourse to practitioners.[33] Much of this practice is adaptive and deserves the support of physicians; some is clearly maladaptive and requires correction. The physician aware of self-care can monitor it and educate patients as to its propriety.

13.   Transference-countertransference reactions occur in many doctor-patient and doctor-family relationships. These reactions are seen most commonly in ongoing relationships, with the physician providing a family with comprehensive care over an extended time period. This is most likely to occur when a member of the family has a chronic illness.

As is now well understood in psychodynamic psychotherapy, patients and family members unconsciously transfer to physicians strong affects associated with early parental childhood experiences. Similarly, physicians do the same. As Balint[29] shows, physicians' unconscious, strong, affective reactions can significantly influence therapeutic relationships in general medical care. "Balint seminars" were designed to enable primary care physicians to systematically examine how these counter-transference reactions can undermine care when anger, fear, or sexual feelings are aroused, and unconsciously brought into play.[29] Family doctors can and should assess and manage these issues routinely.

14.   Stresses caused by the effects of special treatment (e.g., unexpected drug reactions, unavoidable toxicities of chemotherapeutic agents, disfiguring surgeries, highly restrictive diets, therapeutic programs requiring changes in life-style or behavior) represent an important subclass of illness problems. Special treatment environments (e.g., coronary care units, home dialysis, and hospice) may produce predictable stresses for which patients and families need help. If treatment is to be maximized and negative psychosocial consequences minimized, the physician needs to deal with iatrogenic stresses.

It is essential to recognize that treating illness may have undesirable consequences. Reliance on "pop" psychology and common-sense psychotherapy not grounded in appropriate training often results in unsatisfactory outcomes. Sound training in relevant principles can be the best preventative for such misadventures.

CASE STUDY

To facilitate an understanding of the concepts presented in this chapter, a case study is reported. This features elements of psychosocial assessment in primary care.

Biomedical View of the Patient

P. H., a 30-year-old, unemployed, white, married father of two, was admitted to the University Hospital with a two-week history of chills, fever, and malaise. One week prior to admission he visited his LMD with a complaint of "mouth bleeding." Laboratory studies revealed a white blood count of 30,000 and a peripheral blood smear that demonstrated the presence of numerous blast forms. The patient's diagnosis on admission was acute myelogenous leukemia.

The patient's past history, system review, and family history were remarkably negative. He was a heavy user of marijuana. On physical examination, the patient demonstrated scattered petechiae over his body and mucous membranes. His spleen was slightly enlarged. Laboratory studies corroborated the admission diagnosis. The patient was placed on a protocol of chemotherapeutic agents.

The patient's course in the hospital was marked by spiking fevers of 39–40° C. Prophylactic antibiotics were introduced. Because the patient was withdrawn and would not cooperate with the medical staff, a consultation was requested by a team including the authors of this chapter.

Psychosocial Assessment of Patient

This 30-year-old patient, with a diagnosis of acute myelogenous leukemia, has been given a probable prognosis of 2-months without treatment and up to 2 years with treatment. Our consultation service saw him on the request of his medical care team because he was found to be withdrawn, uncooperative, angry, and at times almost combative. Although initially resistant to the consultation team's efforts to interview him, he finally acquiesced, and the following history was obtained. The patient lived in a one-room cabin in rural Washington. He had lived there for the past 6 to 8 years with his wife and two children. The patient said his home was isolated from neighbors. It was without running water and there were outdoor bathroom facilities. About a year earlier, he had held a job as a landscaper for a few months. In general, the family's income had come from his wife's intermittent employment or unemployment insurance. The patient's major activity had been in a motorcycle group with whom he shared marijuana and alcohol.

His family life had been chaotic since youth. His father left him when he was eight years old. The family imposed few limitations on his activities, and his early life was characterized by frequent encounters with the law. His marriage of 9 years was to a woman whose childhood had also been marked by deprivation (an alcoholic father); the marriage was poor in emotional, social, economic, and cultural resources. The patient's commitment to his family had been minimal, but showed some signs of improvement during the past year (occasional expressions of caring for his wife and children, as well as an attempt at employment). He would frequently leave his wife for days at a time without telling her where he was going. Most money was spent on his motorcycle.

At the time the patient was examined by the consultation team, he was depressed, angry, frightened, sick, and ready to give up on life. The consultant team hoped that the psychosocial assessment would answer the question, what does this patient have to live for? We felt that to answer this question, we would need to look at the patient's social support group as well as the explanatory model that he held for his illness.

Social Support Group. The patient's peer group of motorcyclists came to his aid with the offer of blood transfusions; however, they had been infrequent visitors in the hospital. The patient did not focus much of his attention on returning to this group.

The patient's wife, a Jehovah's Witness, indicated that during the years prior to his illness he had experienced some interest in the importance of redemption. There was some consideration, therefore, that religion might play a role in the treatment plan. The patient's wife also gave evidence that her life-style was almost completely family-centered— for better or for worse, she would do all she could to hold her family together. She claimed that she and the children frequently engaged in family activities with members of her religious group.

Patient's Explanatory Model. Guilt did not seem to be an issue in the patient's explanation of why he was ill. The absence of guilt seemed to be in keeping with his past behavior pattern, suggesting a diagnosis of sociopathic character disorder. This diagnosis also seemed to explain, in part, his anger and hostility toward the medical establishment. The patient expressed no clear feeling about the cause of his leukemia. His principal response might best be characterized as "why me?" He saw illness only in individualistic terms. The illness represented a threat and loss to his life, as if he and it were totally separate from his family.

Table 7-2 outlines P. H.'s illness problems that were identified as a result of assessing psychosocial issues. Of interest to the consult group was the macho behavior associated with the motorcycle gang mystique. The message that came through during the patient interview was that members of the motorcycle group were not expected to reveal signs of weakness or ask for help. The patient manifested this behavior by outward signs of resistance, rudeness, not caring, and hostility. Yet, the interview revealed an inner man who seemed lonely, frightened, in pain, and unable to request help because of fears of dependency. The patient seemed to be crying out for someone to break through the angry, rejecting façade. The interpretation made by the consultation team was even though the patient was acting as if he were giving up, he didn't want the medical staff to give up on him. However, his negative transference reaction had provoked many of the staff members to give up. This countertransference response on the part of the staff made the treatment process with this very difficult patient even more vexing, and further alienated the patient.

Discussion

The medical team's biomedical approach to the patient's disease limited their ability to deal with the patient's illness response to a bleak prognosis. The biomedical team confronted the patient with the warning that his noncompliant behavior was fraught with dangers that might result in his earlier demise. Their negotiations were limited to the authoritarian use of the disease model, which the patient predictably met with increased withdrawal and hostility.

The consultation team recommended that by accepting and understanding his perspective of his illness problems and his treatment objectives, therapeutic interventions be negotiated with the patient as a therapeutic ally. In this way, the patient would play an active role in decision-making and would be routinely consulted as a key member of the therapeutic team. The therapeutic plan of the consultants included the following:

1. Identify a physician who would be the primary negotiator.
2. The physician-negotiator's attitude would be one of caring and acceptance even though the patient resisted therapy. This person would demonstrate to the patient that he would stand by him in spite of the patient's rejecting behavior.

TABLE 7-2.   Illness Problems Identified in Patient (P. H.) From Assessment of Psychosocial Issues

Psychosocial Issues Assessed	Patient (P. H.) Illness Problems
1. Coping response	Non-compliant, passive/hostile.
2. Developmental history/ life-cycle (patient's stage of life-cycle, pre-school children)	Limited commitment to family; delinquency; egocentric, irresponsible, and immature behavior.
3. Explanatory model of sickness	Sickness seen in narcissistic terms. Characterized only by "why me?" response.
4. Significance of sickness	Viewed as personal loss or threat of loss.
5. Sociocultural (ethnic) or pre-morbid social role	Anti-authority, anti-establishment, self-serving, motorcycle gang machismo.
6. Patient-health team communication	Resistance to health team's bio-medical-authoritarian approach
7. Family function	Limited commitment to family; however, significant acceptance of patient by family.
8. Labeling sick role	Disabling sickness (patient's role change from active controlling to passive receiving); also, sickness viewed as painful, uncomfortable process.
9. Self-care	Lacks resources to manage disease or illness problems.
10. Transference	Negative response to health care team, who are viewed as authority figures.
11. Countertransference	Health care team responds with anger and withdrawal to patient's non-compliance and threat to their own feelings of efficacy.
12. Special treatment	Secondary effects of chemotherapy (nausea, vomiting, and general malaise) overtly interpreted by patient as being inflicted on him by health care team.
13. Environment	Hospital environment with restriction on mobility and visitations, as well as adherence to routine, contrary to patient's life-style.

3. Negotiations would involve reminding the patient of the support system available to supplement his deficient economic and social resources. The negotiator would clarify for the patient the position of the medical staff, their understanding of his perspective, and outline a treatment regimen that the negotiator believed represented an acceptable compromise on both sides. He would give the patient adequate time to question the plan and help him voice objections and alternatives. The negotiator would then do the same with the medical team and, if needed, the family until a negotiated treatment

contract was hammered out. He would then support the implementation of the plan and monitor compliance of both patient and staff.

4. The physician would encourage a dialogue between husband and wife, so that a measure of mutuality and understanding would develop allowing the couple to cope with their future as a family.

5. Death and dying counseling would be made available to the patient, wife, and children.

6. A meeting would take place with the staff to identify and correct the negative consequences of the patient's transference and the staff's own countertransference. This meeting would emphasize strategies for managing an angry, rejecting patient who protected himself behind an alienating wall of isolation.

Outcome

The patient accepted chemotherapy and remained on the ward for 4 weeks. During this time the physician responsible for the management of the illness problems visited bi-weekly. During these 4 weeks, the medical care team noted a progressive increase in the patient's compliance. Remission of the leukemia occurred and the patient was discharged to his home. One item of encouragement to the consultation team was the patient's expression that he wished to spend his remaining time enjoying his two children.

CONCLUSION

This case history describes an individual who was written off as one who had neither a desire to live nor visible resources. When the biomedical data base was expanded to include a psychosocial assessment, it was found that an understanding of the patient's illness problems offered guidelines for future therapy. Special management strategies were clarified to remedy a deteriorated patient care situation.

This case history was chosen because it represents one of the most difficult problems that a practitioner may encounter. The medical care team had reached an impasse with the patient, the therapeutic atmosphere was demoralized, and both staff and patient were giving up. Attention to the psychosocial issues in primary care assessment was the required element for proper patient management.

REFERENCES

1. Woodruff RA, Goodwin W, Guze SH: *Psychiatric Diagnosis.* New York: Oxford University Press, 1974
2. Nicholi AM (ed): *The Harvard Guide to Modern Psychiatry.* Cambridge, Massachusetts: Harvard University Press, 1978
3. Spritzer RL, Endicott J, Fleiss JL, Cohen J: The psychiatric status schedule and technique for evaluating psychopathology and impairment in role functioning. Arch Gen Psychiatry 23:41–55, 1972
4. Geyman JP: *The Modern Family Doctor and Changing Medical Practice.* New York: Meredith Corporation, 1971
5. Ransom DC, Vandervoort HE: The development of family medicine: Problematic trends. JAMA 225:1,098–102, 1973
6. Shochet BR: Psychological aspects of family practice. Prim Care, 2:93–98, 1975
7. Freedman AN, Kaplan HI, Sadock BJ (eds): *Comprehensive Textbook of Psychiatry.* Baltimore: Williams & Wilkins, 1975
8. Benson DF, Blumer D (eds): *Psychiatric Aspects of Neurological Disease.* New York: Grune and Stratton, 1975
9. Langsley DG, Smilkstein G: "Organic Brain Syndrome." In Rakel RE, Conn HF (eds): *Family Practice.* Philadelphia: W. B. Saunders Company, 1978
10. Engle GL: The need for a new medical model: A challenge for biomedicine. Science 196:129–36, 1977
11. Kleinman A: *Patients and Healers in the Context of Culture: An Exploration of the Borderland between Anthropology, Medicine, and Psychiatry.* Berkeley: University of California Press, 1979
12. Good BJ: The heart of what's the matter: The semantics of illness in Iran. Cul, Med and Psych 1:25–28, 1977
13. Mechanic D: *Medical Sociology.* 2nd ed. New York: Free Press, 1978
14. Kleinman A, Eisenberg K, Good B: Culture, illness and care: Clinical lessons from anthropologic and cross-cultural research. Ann Intern Med 88:251–8, 1978
15. Kleinman A: Relevance for clinical psychiatry and anthropological and cross-cultural research: Concepts and applied strategies. Am J Psychiatry 135:427–31, 1978
16. Moos R: *Coping with Physical Illness.* New York: Plenum Press, 1977
17. Lipowski ZJ: Physical illness, the individual and the coping processes. Psych in Med 1:91–102, 1970
18. Levinson D: *The Seasons of a Man's Life.* New York: Alfred A. Knopf, Inc., 1968
19. Erikson EH: *Childhood and Society.* 2nd ed. New York: Norton, 1963
20. Geyman JP: On growth and development of individuals and families. J Fam Prac 6:739, 1978
21. Medalie JH: *Family Medicine—Principles and Applications.* Baltimore: Williams & Wilkins Company, 1978
22. Chrisman N, Kleinman A: "Health Beliefs of American Ethnic Groups." *Harvard Encyclopedia of American Ethnic Groups.* Cambridge, Mass: Harvard University Press, in press

23. Snow L: Folk medicine beliefs and their implications for care of patients. Ann Intern Med 81:82–96, 1974

24. Fabrega H, Manning PK: An integrated theory of disease: Ladino-Mestizo views of disease in the Chiapas highlands. Psychosom Med 35:223–239, 1973

25. Harwood A: The hot-cold theory of disease: Implications for treatment of Puerto Rican patients. JAMA 216:1,153–60, 1971

26. Bertakis KD: The communication of information from physician to patient: A method for increasing patient retention and satisfaction. J Fam Prac 5:217–22, 1977

27. Kleinman A: "Explanatory Models in Health Care Relationship." In *Health of the Family.* Washington, D.C.: National Council for International Health, 1975

28. Svarstad B: "Physician-Patient Communications and Patient Conformity with Medical Advice." In Mechanic D: *The Growth of Bureaucratic Medicine.* New York: Wiley Interscience Publications, 159–172, 1976

29. Balint M: *The Doctor, His Patient and the Illness.* New York: International Universities Press, 1957

30. Twaddle AC: Concepts of health status. Soc Sci Med 8:29–38, 1974

31. Kane R, et al: Manipulating the patient: A comparison of the effectiveness of physicians and chiropractic care. 1:1,333–36, 1974

32. Cay EL, et al: Patient assessment of the result of surgery for peptic ulcer. Lancet 1:29–31, 1975

33. Kleinman A: International health care planning from an ethnomedical perspective: Critique and recommendations for change. Med Anthro 2:71–96, 1978

CHAPTER 8

BASIC INTERVIEWING SKILLS

CHARLES KENT SMITH AND JOHN H. LEVERSEE

Since the medical interview is the basis for almost all patient contact by the family physician, it is of great importance that the principles of interviewing be understood in some detail. In this chapter, the medical interview will be analyzed and broken down into discrete parts which may then be taught and learned.

INTRODUCTION

Effective medical interviewing is not just a conversation, it is a learned skill. Osler is reputed to have said: "If you take a history and you don't know what is wrong with the patient, go back and take another history." Many authorities place the value of the medical history at 80 to 90 percent of any patient evaluation. Some physicians are able to obtain essential, accurate data in a short time while others find it a struggle and miss much essential material. This certainly is a common clinical observation and has been studied in a variety of situations. In their book, *Doctors Talking To Patients,* Byrne and Long[1] have analyzed the verbal interactions of a large number of general practitioners in their consultations

109

with approximately 2500 patients over a 3½-year period. They noted that doctors are both the product and prisoner of a training system that has emphasized organic disease and created a variety of sins of omission and commission. The reader further interested in the interview process is referred to this book. The point of this and other studies is that increased competence in the medical interview will lead to more accurate diagnosis and treatment of both medical and psychosocial problems. Skillfully done, interviewing saves the physician and the patient valuable time and allows the physician to render the best possible care.

SETTING AND EXTERNAL FACTORS

Careful attention must be paid to the setting of the interview and other external factors affecting communication. The patient will probably be most comfortable and the interview most successful if the patient and doctor are alone, either in the doctor's office or in the hospital setting. This is often a problem in the hospital where there are two or more patients in a room. It may be appropriate to take the patient to an examining room or consultation room where privacy is assured. Or perhaps the roommate can be asked to go to the lounge if his or her condition allows for easier ambulation. With the hospitalized patient, avoid interviewing after sedation or narcotic medication. Avoid mealtimes, bedpan times, and nurse interruptions. Nurses should be informed when an interview will take place.

There should be adequate lighting, neither too bright, nor too dark. It is helpful not to have the light source directly behind the physician or the patient; this tends to establish one or the other as dominant.

There should be satisfactory noise control. The patient who hears voices from the next room will realize that the interview can be overheard, and this may limit the depth or accuracy of the communication. The radio or television should be turned off. It is ludicrous to attempt a medical interview while the patient's eyes are glued to a television screen.

Whenever possible, the setting should be arranged so that the physician is at eye level with the patient. In this way neither is set up to be dominant. The physician may direct and lead the interview but, by truly dominating the situation, valuable communication may be lost. On hospital rounds, the physician should take time to sit by the patient's bedside, thus appearing unhurried. This also allows eyelevel contact with the patient. A short period of time spent in this manner will be interpreted by the patient to be longer and more personal than an extended period of time spent standing at the bedside looking at (and talking down to) the patient. More information will be obtained and it will probably be more accurate and more meaningful.

NOTE-TAKING

This can be an individual matter. Most patients are not bothered by note-taking if it is done discretely and without overemphasis. In fact, note-taking will often reassure patients that what they have to say is important. This applies particularly to factual and more clearly "medical" information. When discussing more personal and emotionally laden information it is often useful to put down the pen and listen more intently.

It is also useful to discuss note-taking with the patient and what goes in the medical record. The same is true for forms. If the patient understands the purpose of forms, the written information can extend what is learned from the interview.

OPENING THE INTERVIEW

It has been said that the essence of a good doctor-patient relationship is to be warm, interested, understanding, and nonjudgmental. These qualities should be kept in mind when starting an interview with the patient.

If the physician and patient are meeting for the first time, there should be an introduction. It is important to listen for the patient's name and understand the proper pronounciation. It is also a good idea to clear up any questions about family relationships with other patients. For example, "you are Betty Jones' sister." It is a common courtesy to let patients know that the doctor is pleased to see them. This is facilitated by establishing eye contact, thus presenting a pleasant appearance. Too many physicians appear to be aloof and preoccupied.

As soon as it is convenient, perhaps on subsequent meetings, come to an agreement about the use of first names. Some patients like to be called by their first name and still refer to the physician as doctor. However, it is becoming more common that patients do not always want their first names used. If a patient's first name is used, this sets up the expectation that the physician's first name may be used in return, which may or may not produce discomfort for the physician. This resolution is unimportant, as long as both physician and patient are comfortable and there has been mutual agreement.

Next, it is important that both physician and patient are clear as to the purpose of the interview. It is disconcerting to launch into a history for a complete examination when the patient is there with a minor problem for a brief office visit. Of course, the reverse is just as upsetting. It is preferable to ask early in the interview why the patient is there and what is expected during that visit. When time is limited, the physician should state the length of time that has been planned. The patient can then turn to priority items promptly and save less important things for another appointment. Clear understanding of the problems to be dealt with and the expected time frame can avoid misunderstandings and unreal expectations on the part of both physician and patient. Of course, unexpected things may arise throwing the best-laid plans awry, but most of the time the above will prove very beneficial.

CLOSING THE INTERVIEW

It is advantageous for both the patient and the physician to have a definite close to the interview. Be sure the patient knows the visit is over and the physician will not be coming back into the room. Ideally, the patient may be asked if there are any other questions or if there is anything further to say. Patients will then be more likely to feel their needs have been met and will be content to end the interview. If this is not the case, the physician may need to be quite assertive and state that the session is over. This is best handled by informing the patient that the other items will be addressed on another visit. It also creates a good feeling if patients are told that the physician enjoyed the interview and appreciates the opportunity to provide for their care.

WHAT THE PHYSICIAN AND PATIENT BRING

Everyone brings a lifetime of prior experience to every encounter with another human being. Personalities are shaped first by one's family and later by peers, teachers, clergymen, and others who are part of one's life.

Each person carries multiple memories and experiences, as well as feelings, emotions, opinions, and prejudices. A person is conscious of many of these, but not all. Two main concepts deriving from a psychodynamic approach to psychosocial development are pertinent to the interviewing situation.[2] One concerns defense mechanisms and the other deals with transference.

Defense mechanisms have become part of common parlance, for example: denial, repression, and reaction formation.[3] A basic understanding of psychological development also gives some appreciation of different personality styles such as the angry, compulsive, or dependent person.[4]

Another concept from the psychodynamic framework that is important to the interview is that of transference. Briefly, this means that persons important in one's early life, especially but not exclusively parents, leave a legacy of opinions, feelings, and emotions. These feelings may not be in conscious awareness, but in some form they will be transferred to others, particularly those with whom one deals closely. In its simplest form an example might be a male physician who evokes the same kind of response and reactions the patient had to his own father. The other side of this coin is that the physician has gone through his own development and has multiple unconscious ideas and feelings that will affect reactions to the patient.

Reactions toward individuals and groups or classes of people will also be influenced by one's prejudices. Religious, ethical, sexual, and social differences may have effects in a variety of ways. Understanding one's own prejudices can enable the physician to be better accepting, open, and nonjudgmental—all important features for a successful medical interview.

THE INTERVIEW ITSELF

Observation

Although it seems that close observation of the patient is done automatically, it is not. How many times has a patient left the consultation room uncertain whether a lesion was on the right side or the left, or on which quadrant of the abdomen a scar was located? A great deal of information is available if the physician is trained for observation. Consider the classic observation by Sherlock Holmes in *Silver Blaze.*

> **HOLMES:**
> *I would like to call to your attention the curious incident of the dog in the night time.*
>
> **INSPECTOR GREGORY:**
> *The dog did nothing in the night time.*
>
> **HOLMES:**
> *That was the curious incident.*

What is the patient's general appearance, body habitus, speech pattern, memory, and orientation? Is the patient's affect appropriate; what is the patient's mood? Can the patient understand what the physician is saying and answer appropriately? These should all be looked for and noted.

Nonverbal Communication

A great deal of information is communicated nonverbally. Persons consciously and unconsciously express themselves and receive messages from others through body language. The physician needs to be alert for situations in which the patient's expression or body language is conveying a different message than the one being verbalized.

In certain examinations, such as an injury-illness situation, it can be very comforting and reassuring if the physician will touch the patient. This can be a hand on the patient's shoulder or arm during a routine examination, a gentle touch on the injured area, or provision of support to an injured extremity. The attitude of caring expressed by this closeness and touching can help the physician establish what has been called the essence of a good doctor-patient relationship; warmth, interest, understanding, and a nonjudgmental attitude.

It is possible for the same attitude to prevail in the interview situation. The skilled physician will choose when to treat the patient in a manner that is a verbal and postural equivalent of reaching out and "touching." The following are ways of increasing those aspects of communication:

1.   Posture. Chances for good communication increase when one sits or stands comfortably, avoiding a tense and anxious position. The physician should not sit rigidly on the chair or lounge away from the patient. Arms and legs should not be crossed, fists clenched, or hands covering part of the face. The physician should be at eye level with the patient, if possible. A distance that is comfortably acceptable should be maintained. Cultural variations are important to consider; Latin-American patients or those from Arab countries may prefer a closeness that is uncomfortable for Americans. In the United States, the usually acceptable separation between doctor and patient is 2½ to 3 feet. A position should be found that is most comfortable for both parties.

2.   General Appearance. The physician should wear clean, well kept, appropriate dress. A doctor's coat may or may not help communication. Consider the impact of other medical symbols such as a stethoscope, reflex hammer, or the chart. These items may intimidate some patients.

3.   Facial Expressions. Eye contact should be maintained as much as possible. When appropriate the physician should smile. The patient's eyes and facial expressions should be observed as the interview progresses.

4.   Hands. Hands can often be very expressive. The physician should not clasp them or make a fist. The patient's hands should be observable.

QUESTIONING

1.   Open-ended Questions. An open-ended question is broad in scope and does not limit or do more than roughly define the area of inquiry. Open-ended questions allow the patient the greatest possible latitude in

answering. The patient then identifies the elements of an illness that require discussion. Thus, the patient's answer may be in the realm of physical complaints, the emotional sphere, or, of course, any area. The patient has the freedom to communicate a problem without any bias introduced by a particular line of questioning. Examples: "Tell me about your illness," "What brought you in today?" or "I would like to hear (or know) more about your family." The importance of open-ended questions cannot be overemphasized.

2.   Focused Questions. With focused questions the interviewer defines the area of inquiry, but allows the patient considerable latitude in answering. For example: "Describe the chest pain." Two general areas have been focused upon: a symptom, the pain, and a region of the body, the chest. The patient will then confine further responses to these areas.

3.   Closed Questions. These are questions that can be answered by yes or no or by a numerical answer, such as age, number of children, times per day. Other examples are questions that pinpoint a specific date, day, time, place, or person's name. The information is limited but may be very important.

4.   Leading Questions. The interviewer suggests an answer to his own question. Implicit in this is a bias, value, or a wish held by the interviewer. Example: "You are feeling better, aren't you?"

5.   Compound Questions. The interviewer may ask two or more questions without giving the patient time to respond. Another example is a string of separate questions, or one question that asks for a multicomponent response.

Leading and compound questions are defined for purposes of clarification and condemnation; they should not be used!

The following diagram depicts the amount of information obtainable from different types of questioning:

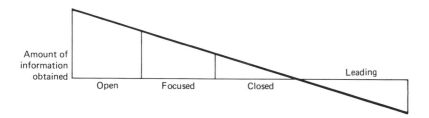

It is most productive to start interviews with open-ended questions and then move to focused and closed-questions. Many times most of the needed information will come from the open-ended questions. With a rambling patient, it is necessary to be more focused and direct. Leading and compound questions should always be avoided.

LISTENING-RESPONDING SKILLS

Listening and responding skills are as important and difficult to master as questioning skills. Physicians are most used to "doing something," so that actually listening to what the patient is trying to say is generally more difficult. It is important to realize that active listening is doing something! Good listening and responding techniques let the patient know that the physician has heard what was said and what was meant. The specific skills in this area follow:

1. Confirmation. This response reassures the patient that the physician is listening and encourages the patient to continue. For example: "Okay," "All right," "I understand," or even "Uh huh."

2. Silence. Anything passive is hard for physicians, particularly if they are uncomfortable or unsure of themselves in a given area. Many physicians have the compulsion to jump in and help the patient; yet silence is a critical listening skill. A well-known psychiatrist is rumored to have said that an entire psychoanalysis could be conducted without the psychiatrist saying a word. Although this is apocryphal and certainly not in the interest of good human relationships, it is nevertheless indicative of the value of silence. Silence encourages patients to speak what is truly on their mind.

When the patient has said something that is hard to believe, made a weak defense for his action, transferred blame, or otherwise made the physician feel a need to contradict, challenge, or confront, a short period of contemplative silence on the part of the physician can allow the patient to reassess and modify the statement. The skill to not speak at such times is distinctly not easy to master.

3. Empathy. In this mode the interviewer labels as accurately as possible the emotion the patient felt or is feeling. This differs from paraphrasing for the physician is identifying the emotional state or feeling, not just the historical content or factual information. When the patient reveals something emotionally important, it is very reassuring to know the physician recognizes the feeling. For example:

PATIENT:
I didn't know what to think this morning. When I woke up, I couldn't feel anything from my elbow to my fingertips.

PHYSICIAN:
That must have been frightening for you.

4. Summary. It is often helpful for the physician to briefly summarize the patient's report, adopting what is believed to be the patient's point of view. This is especially true at the conclusion of a lengthy, con-

fusing or disjointed account; the physician's summary should then verify the important events and relationships. When an area appears sufficiently investigated, a summary may allow the physician and patient to move comfortably to a new topic.

Summarizing communicates to the patient the physician's interest in an accurate understanding of the events that the patient has related. Conversely, inaccurate summaries tell the patient that the physician has not listened carefully or has received inaccurate information. Summaries require hard work, but they provide useful feedback on the physician's ability to listen.

5. Confrontation. This technique is used frequently in a psychiatric interviewing situation. Confrontation means making an observation about the patient's behavior, appearance, or a story which has been withheld. This often implies or explicitly recognizes a discrepancy or need for more information. For example: "You say you have a close family unit, but you have not told me anything about your children" or "You've told me you like your job, but you look very discouraged whenever you talk about it." Confrontation does *not* mean making hostile, accusatory, or pejorative remarks to the patient. It does not imply that the patient has been caught or trapped in a mistake. In the best sense, it provides the patient with a certain amount of insight and it directs attention to something of which the patient may not have been aware.

6. Restatement or Clarification. With restatement the physician briefly repeats something that has just been said. Clarification may involve a restatement, but here the physician asks the patients to help further define what was meant. Patients will almost invariably respond by elaborating on the points the physician wishes to pursue. For example:

PATIENT:
To tell you the truth, doctor, I am not at all well.

PHYSICIAN:
Not at all well?

7. Interpretation. A rephrasing of the patient's statements in the physician's own words, an inference, or synthesizing information from the physician's own perspective are all examples of interpretation.

PATIENT:
My children check up on me a lot when I'm at home. They seem to enjoy dropping by. And, they take turns visiting me at the hospital.

PHYSICIAN:
It sounds like you have a close-knit family.

If the physician continually parrots what the patient has said, it may not be helpful and may be an irritant. This is not the purpose of interpretation.

Interpretation should rarely be done at an early phase of an interview. It is most appropriately saved until the end, preferably when some sort of reliable doctor-patient relationship has been established.

ACTIVE LISTENING

The term, "Active Listening," has been coined by Thomas Gordon[5] and encompasses several valuable skills in the interview situation. Careful attention is paid to the verbal and nonverbal real message a patient expresses. Factual information is carefully collated, and the interview continues until the physician is certain of the message being transmitted. At this point, the message is reflected back to the patient as accurately as possible. This response is akin to, but goes further than, empathy. The patient is assured that the physician really heard and understood the feelings expressed.

The real meaning or feeling of a message may come more from how something is said, or the body language that accompanies the statement, than from the statement itself. An easy message to interpret would be the patient who answers "just fine," but has a lowered voice and downcast eyes. In such a case one would most likely follow with, "It doesn't look as though things are so fine. Tell me how you really feel." Somewhat harder messages to interpret are those of fear or concern. Patients may ask if a certain procedure is "really necessary" or could a test or operation be delayed for a period of time. That patient will be much more satisfied with an answer such as, "It seems as though you are frightened (or concerned). Let's talk about this some more." That is active listening and means much more to the patient than, "You have nothing to worry about," or "You don't need to worry, I'll do the worrying for you." The patient has just indicated worry and it does not help to be told not to worry. After the physician acknowledges the patient's fears, then an explanation of the low risks of the procedure will have a much more receptive audience.

SPECIAL CONSIDERATIONS IN COMMUNICATION

One approach to the analysis of communication is to consider the patient as the sender of information, and the physician as the receiver and interpreter.

Appropriate use of the information requires a differentiation between a "condition" and a "problem." A condition can be a diagnosis such as hypertension, a measurement such as weight or blood pressure, an observation of behavior such as smoking, and other similar conditions. A problem is something that the patient perceives as a problem.

The physician's goal is to discover what conditions are present and then to determine which are problems to the patient. This does not mean that a condition holding potential danger to a patient's health should not be dealt with; but there may be difficulty establishing a therapeutic regimen until the patient perceives it as a problem. In this regard, it is helpful to include in the interview some questions such as the following:

Is this a problem for you?
How is that a problem for you?
Can you conceive of this condition becoming a problem for you?

A classic example of a misunderstanding between a condition and a problem occurred with a hospitalized patient. A 56-year-old diabetic woman was hospitalized because of moderately severe ketoacidosis. She had stopped taking her insulin about 2 weeks prior to admission and gave no clear reason for her action. In the hospital, her behavior was judged to be difficult and recalcitrant. She frequently discarded urines before they were checked for sugar and ketone, and she did not keep a record of intake and output. The physicians became angry and frustrated. They were directing a great deal of effort and expertise toward balancing her diabetes, but there was clearly poor doctor-patient communication, and lack of compliance with treatment plans. One morning when there was time to inquire in an open-ended manner "How are things going?" they discovered that the patient's principal concern was lower extremity pain, particularly in the hips and knees. This pain had been present for nearly 6 months. During office visits and this hospitalization, her doctor's attention was always directed to her diabetes, which was *assumed* to be her major problem; yet, it was this pain that had been preventing housework, shopping and recreation. Perhaps in frustration or in an attempt to have more contact with her doctors, she had been noncompliant regarding her diabetic care. After pursuing a careful history of the lower extremity pain, she said: "Thank goodness someone is talking to me about my pain." After further investigation, she was started on treatment for polymyalgia rheumatica. Her behavior changed dramatically. She was compliant regarding her diabetic care, and she conversed easily with all members of the health care team.

INTERVIEWING FOR THE SEXUAL HISTORY

The importance of this chapter is highlighted when consideration is given to difficult content areas such as sexuality. Obtaining a sexual history is a part of basic interviewing, yet it is a task with which many physicians are not yet comfortable.

Regarding sexuality in the United States, the thought has been expressed that we are (1) ignorant, (2) traumatized, and (3) secretive. If this is the case, it is no wonder that obtaining a sexual history is initially difficult for patient and physician.

A comfortable interview on sexual topics can be accomplished if the physician develops the necessary skills, maintains a nonjudgmental attitude, and has a conviction that sexuality is an important area in the patient's total health. It is helpful to be nonthreatening and to ask tangential questions before proceeding to more difficult areas. The sexual history may be commenced by asking a fairly open question such as: "How have things been going in your marriage (relationship)?" or "Do you feel you made a good choice?" After these questions have been answered and discussed, one could ask: "How has the sexual portion of your marriage worked out?" With young teenagers, one might ask: "How were your school health education classes? Did they do a good job of teaching about sex?" Next would come the question: "If you decided to be sexually active, do you have enough knowledge to protect yourself from pregnancy and VD?"

These approaches allow the patient to discuss elements in his or her sexual history without feeling threatened or exposed. Most patients desire to talk about aspects of their sexual lives and will do so, if given the proper opportunity. There are times when it is especially important to take a sexual history. Examples would be:

1. Where a full history and physical is being done.
2. When the patient presents with an overt sexual problem.
3. When an organic disease demands attention to the area.
4. When a sexual problem is suspected to be involved with the patient's problem, although it may not be apparent.

In our society, a physician is often perceived to be the most nonthreatening and knowledgeable person the patient can talk to about his sexual life. It is therefore incumbent upon physicians to develop the necessary skills and attitudes to facilitate obtaining a sexual history.[6]

RECENT LITERATURE ON INTERVIEWING

Many good recent texts on interviewing have appeared in the last few years, often with an orientation toward the primary care physician. Books by Froelich and Bishop,[7] Enelow and Swisher,[8] and Benjamin,[9] are all useful as are chapters in recent family medicine texts, such as that by

Rakel.[10] We have referred to the monograph by Byrne,[1] which provides a rich variety of observations on the interview.

Studies have been carried out on verbal and nonverbal aspects of the interview in a family medicine setting.[11] Videotaped interviews with physicians in training and experienced physicians were carefully analyzed, making observations every 15 seconds, using some standardized interactional models. The study was done in the context of relating interview behavior with patient satisfaction and understanding of the encounter with the physician. Patient satisfaction was found to be associated significantly with informing, or explaining. Patient understanding of the interview was correlated with summarizing, empathetic responses, as well as with informing and explaining. Satisfaction was negatively correlated when closed or compound questions were asked. Closer distances with the patient were associated with higher satisfaction and understanding. The amount of time spent with the patient was significant; longer periods correlated with higher satisfaction and understanding.

In summary, interviewing is a learned skill. Identification of component skills is the first step in the development of good interviewing techniques.

REFERENCES

1. Byrne PS, Long B: *Doctors Talking to Patients.* St. Allen's, Campfield Press, For Her Majesty's Stationery Office, 1976
2. Freedman AM, Kaplan HI, Sadock BJ: *Modern Synopsis of Comprehensive Textbook of Psychiatry II.* Baltimore: Williams & Wilkins, 1976
3. Freud A: *The Ego and The Mechanism of Defense.* Translated by Cecil Baines. New York: International Universities Press, 1946
4. Lipp M: *Respectful Treatment.* Hagerstown, Md: Harper & Row, 1977
5. Gordon T: *Parent Effectiveness Training.* New York: Peter H. Wyden, Inc, 1970
6. Masters WH, Johnson V: *Human Sexual Inadequacy.* Boston: Little, Brown & Co., 1970
7. Froelich RE, Bishop FM: *Clinical Interviewing Skills.* St. Louis: The C. V. Mosby Company, 1977
8. Enelow AJ, Swisher SN: *Interviewing and Patient Care.* New York: Oxford University Press, 1972
9. Benjamin A: *The Helping Interview.* Boston: Houghton Mifflin Co., 1969
10. Rakel R: *Principles of Family Medicine.* Philadelphia: W. B. Saunders Co, 1977
11. Smith CK, Polis E: *Characteristics of the Initial Interview for Patient Satisfaction and Understanding.* 1979, Presented at the North America Primary Care Research Group, Toronto, Canada (April, 1978)

CHAPTER 9

INTERVIEWING THE DIFFICULT PATIENT

DAVID D. SCHMIDT AND EDWARD MESSNER

INTRODUCTION

The techniques described in this chapter are appropriate for certain specific patients or situations in which it can be anticipated that an interview will present some difficulty for the family physician. It will be assumed that the physician has attained facility in talking with patients under more ordinary circumstances. In order to establish a foundation from which later sections can expand, a brief outline of a general interview in a medical setting is included in this introduction.

In the opening moments of an encounter with a patient—particularly a new patient—the physician should try to facilitate a warm, natural introduction. A few moments of small talk on a topic of interest to the patient helps to establish a comfortable atmosphere. The actual interview is best begun with open-ended questions such as, "What can I do for you today?" or "What brings you to the office?"* As the story begins to unfold, one must demonstrate a respectful concern about the patient's

* Other examples: "Tell me what has been happening." "What has been going on?" "What has been affecting you?"

complaint or problem, no matter how trivial it may appear. Trivia often serve as decoys or disguises. Give the patient time to complete his or her narration. A hurried appearance or show of impatience may inhibit communication.

Although the interview begins with open-ended questions, the physician will eventually want to obtain more specific information appropriate to the particular problem. This should be explained to the patient. Make every effort to avoid firing question after question in a threatening fashion that might appear to the patient to be an inquisition. One must always remain sensitive to the patient's reactions, both verbal and nonverbal, to a particular line of questioning. Consider another means of obtaining the same material, if one approach is making the patient uncomfortable. If one must continue in sensitive areas, stop and take the time to explain why you believe this information will be helpful in the solution of the patient's problems. Whenever the patient appears puzzled, provide some feedback, and explanation. This will serve to enhance trust and confidence.

One should probe gently for underlying fears that may accompany the complaint. Helping the patient to be more explicit about these concerns makes the physician's resources more effective to alleviate such fears. In a medical setting, this may include the physical examination and laboratory evaluation (such as the examination of a lipoma of the skin feared to be cancer, or a hematocrit in the patient who thought she was tired because of "low blood"). In a counseling situation, simple reassurance (such as fear of mental retardation because of masturbation) can be most effective. In a more complex psychotherapeutic effort, the expression of hidden fears frequently marks the beginning of a desirable change.

Physicians should always be sensitive to the quality of communication between themselves and their patients. The physician should avoid using medical jargon or language that the patient does not understand. There should be a warm and gentle, nonjudgmental and accepting attitude, rather than one that is distant, harsh, judgmental, and patronizing. The physician should strive to pick up and adequately pursue symptoms or feelings mentioned casually by the patient. In the concluding moments of the encounter, the physician ought to make an effort to summarize the problems discussed and form a clear plan for future management. An explicit contract should be established with the patient. In the final few moments, another opportunity must be provided for the patient to express concerns. Frequently, the "by-the-way" comments are the most revealing.

Table 9-1 is a list of common psychosocial problems encountered in family practice. This is not meant to be all-inclusive. Patients with these

TABLE 9-1.   Common Psychosocial Problems

1. Anxiety states
2. Depression
3. Sexual malfunction
4. Disturbed family relationship and family counseling
5. Alcoholism and drug abuse
6. Emotional problems that accompany acute and chronic illness or death
7. Geriatric problems and emotional needs of the elderly
8. Personality disorders
9. Adjustment reaction of adolescence

conditions are frequently under considerable stress, which interferes with their ability to communicate with others, including health professionals. We plan to discuss the nature of the communication difficulties associated with five of these nine problems to offer some interviewing techniques that may be helpful for each situation. We hope the approach of using concrete examples helps the reader to gain new insights into the techniques of interviewing "difficult" patients.

Another means of classifying the difficult patient would be in terms of the emotional state which interferes with communication. This includes a listing such as the angry patient, the sad patient, or the frightened patient. We encourage the physician to try to define the problem in more detail. This additional effort greatly facilitates the interviewing process, and is a prerequisite for any therapeutic effort.

A patient may be angry because of a basic personality disorder, sad because of a depressive reaction, or frightened following a hyperventilation episode. Any sensitive layman can appreciate another's emotional state. A skillful professional will ask the question: "Why is the patient angry, sad, or frightened?" Communication begins with the physician's sensitive search for the answer.

ANXIETY REACTION

The example discussed of an acute anxiety reaction is the hyperventilation syndrome. When the patient with hyperventilation is seen during an acute episode, this condition is readily recognized. In the extreme form, the patient is exceedingly anxious and terrified, gasping for air, complaining of light-headedness and paresthesia in the extremities and around the mouth. At times, carpal-pedal spasm may be seen. In this acute situation, having the patient breathe into a paper bag to recirculate carbon dioxide will end the episode. Relatively few individuals are seen during such an acute episode. The physician is more commonly consulted within a few hours or days, at which time the diagnosis is less obvious. This problem is seen more frequently in females than in males.

As the patient describes symptoms, and the physician begins to appreciate their psychosomatic origin, extreme care must be taken not to dismiss these symptoms as trivial or unimportant. The symptoms are very real, and extremely frightening for the patient. Furthermore, as the physician proceeds to explain and reassure, the message that it's "all in your head" must be avoided. It may be helpful to explain that anyone would experience the same symptoms as a result of hyperventilation. Another common feature is that the patient may not appreciate that breathing was faster than normal. Explaining that a few extra breaths per minute, continued over a long period of time, produces the same effect as extreme hyperventilation over shorter periods of time, may lend more credibility to the explanation. Finally, demonstrating that the symptoms are produced by voluntary hyperventilation appears most convincing to the patient. An explanation of the physiology involved, expressed in simple, understandable terms, further helps to emphasize that the patient does not have a serious underlying disease.

Once the patient has accepted this explanation, the physician should proceed by saying something like, "In most cases of hyperventilation, some sort of tension, worry, or anxiety seems to trigger the rapid breathing; do you believe that this is the situation in your case?" or, "Are you struggling with any particular problems, worries, or tensions?" If this gentle exploration uncovers a problem, it should be explored in some depth. If, on the other hand, the patient is unable to identify a reason for being anxious, ask the patient to explore the possibilities with his family, and try to be observant of the initiating events or concerns should such an episode return.

In many instances, the appearance of the hyperventilation syndrome represents a reaction to an acute, stressful event. In this situation, simple reassurance is often therapeutic. This syndrome may also be indicative of a serious or chronic underlying psychological problem requiring a more intensive psychotherapeutic effort, perhaps psychotherapy. The basic principle underlying the management of the former situation is the physician's calm and concerned clarification of the relationship between the stress and the syndrome. This should include an explanation emphasizing that the patient is experiencing a normal physiologic reaction. It is important to state explicitly that there is no underlying disease, particularly in the lungs and heart. Fear of the unknown increases the level of anxiety. Confident recognition of the symptoms and a positive explanation by the physician can be quite therapeutic.

Following this initial effort at reassurance, the patient should be given at least one follow-up appointment. At the return visit, the physician can assess the need for further evaluation of the psychosocial problems.

DEPRESSION

Anxiety and depression are frequently encountered together in the same patient. The illustrative case history demonstrates that by simply developing a family history and family tree, a great deal of significant psychosocial information can be obtained during a medical encounter. Finally, some suggested areas for exploration in interviews with depressed patients are discussed.

Case Presentation

This 33-year-old female was first seen on January 30, 1978, complaining of episodes of light-headedness, shortness of breath, and paresthesia in all four extremities. Her physical examination was not remarkable, and voluntary hyperventilation reproduced her symptoms. She fully appreciated that she had been experiencing considerable stress by trying to hold down two jobs and rearing a 7-year-old son by herself. The physician's reassurance provided some initial improvement. Ten days later she was seen as a "walk-in" because of "tightness" in her chest and a pounding heart. Physical examination was unremarkable, and an ECG was within normal limits.

The next day she came into the office accompanied by her brother. They both strongly urged hospitalization. Although she was still having episodes of anxiety, the vegetative signs of depression began to dominate the clinical picture. She became quite tearful, experienced early morning awakening, and had lost her appetite. Further questioning revealed that she had lost a total of 10 lbs. in the past several weeks. She had not been working regularly, and her 7-year-old son was temporarily staying with the grandparents. At this point, she agreed to return for a scheduled appointment which provided adequate time for a more complete history and medical evaluation.

In the course of developing the family tree, diagrammed in Figure 9-1, the following information was obtained. The patient is the seventh of nine children. Her mother is 64 years old with many medical problems. The patient married her late husband 12 years ago. Two years after the marriage, there was a full-term stillbirth of a female fetus. The second child of this marriage is currently 7 years old. Her husband was the only child of a 45-year-old mother in good health, and a 52-year-old father.

In 1975, the patient and her husband were having some marital difficulties. They were separated, and the husband moved to Atlanta. The patient did not know his whereabouts. The husband's parents would fly

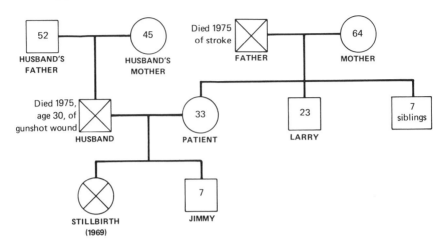

FIGURE 9-1.   Family tree of patient—1978.

the grandson to Atlanta for periodic visits with the father, but shielded his location from the patient. After being separated for three months, the husband was shot and killed by a friend in an argument. His parents have successfully concealed the circumstances of this killing. They also took care of all the funeral arrangements. Three months later, the patient's father died of a stroke.

The patient feels that her father-in-law is supportive, but that her mother-in-law is disparaging of her ability to raise the young boy. The patient has made a special effort to allow the ex-husband's parents access to their grandson. She has the distinct impression that her ex-husband's parents hold her partially responsible for their son's death, and is very fearful that the grandparents will take her son away from her.

The medical evaluation failed to reveal any physical cause for the patient's symptoms, and she agreed to explore the emotional problems further. How does one proceed from this point?

The family history provides many clues for structuring future interviews that might prove most productive. The first question is why has the patient become depressed at this particular moment in time; what precipitated the depression? She managed to cope with many major crises in the past. If the answer to this question is not readily apparent, the possibility of a beginning psychosis, an affective disorder, or other psychiatric condition must be considered. Careful attention to mental status examination, and an alertness for possible thought disturbance would be indicated.

A significant loss, real or imagined, is frequently associated with a depressive reaction. Within recent years, this patient had a stillborn child,

her father died, and she lost her husband by a sudden and violent death during a period of marital disharmony. The feelings surrounding each of these losses should be explored. An unresolved grief reaction combined with her inability to maintain two jobs might explain the depression and a probable loss of self esteem.

Guilt is another dynamic often presented in depressed patients. Does she harbor any guilt for the death of the fetus, or believe that the marital disharmony created circumstances ending in her husband's death? Is there any element of guilt in the grief reaction to her father's death?

Most experienced family physicians can easily recognize the depressed patient with somatic complaints. It can be more difficult to proceed with interviews that uncover the cause of the depression. This diagnostic effort frequently becomes therapeutic for the patient if the exploration leads to greater insights. Searches for a precipitating cause, real or imagined loss, and feelings of guilt are specific ways to begin this process.

In this specific case, it was eventually learned that when the patient first developed somatic complaints and sought medical care, she was becoming heavily involved with a male friend who was making sexual demands. This experience awakened her memories of the conflicts she had had with her husband and the circumstances that surrounded his death.

DISTURBED FAMILY RELATIONSHIP AND FAMILY COUNSELING

The example to be discussed under this category is the family crisis of impending divorce. The family physician is in a unique position to help during such a crisis. Since the physician may have performed the premarital examinations, cared for both the man and woman during episodes of illness, and been entrusted with the health supervision of their children, the couple often turn to their physician for help during a difficult period. The troubled couple may seek out the family physician early if a willingness to help with interpersonal problems has been demonstrated (perhaps at the time of the premarital examinations).

Often, one partner (usually the man) is reluctant to seek help from a psychiatrist or marriage counselor. The psychiatrist is someone outside the ordinary experience of most people, and is as remote as the radiologist or pathologist. In contrast, almost everyone has turned to a general medical doctor for help at one time or another. On rare occasions, the close relationship with the family physician may make it difficult for a patient to discuss painful subjects, such as infidelity. In such instances, the physician should recognize the necessity of finding another source of help.

When a practicing family physician is confronted with a marital crisis, there are three choices: ignore the plea for help, refer the couple to another source for marriage counseling, or deal with the problem directly. If immediate referral is chosen, the physician risks engendering a feeling of rejection in the couple who had finally developed courage to discuss their problem. In addition, it is well known that a large percentage of these patients will not accept the referral.

To be effective in obtaining potentially painful information, the physician must take a neutral stance. It is necessary to clearly demonstrate that the physician's major role is to help them understand why they are having problems and to aid them in finding possible solutions. This is accomplished by rational discussion facilitated by the physician referee. This neutral position can be enhanced by having the physician first talk to both parties individually, followed by a few sessions together. At the onset of this counseling effort, the physician and the couple should agree to devote four to six sessions of 30 to 40 minutes each. An effort involving less time will probably not be helpful.

Only after individuals are able to talk openly with one another about their feelings can any progress be expected. The physician must be comfortable with discussing the couple's sexual relationship and, equally important, must have a thorough knowledge of human sexuality. The physician must have sufficient psychiatric background to recognize major neurotic problems or personality disorders when they exist and, as with all fields of medicine, must recognize his or her limitations and seek psychiatric consultation when appropriate.

The family physician can make a significant contribution to the quality of family life, particularly when the husband and wife are basically healthy and free of major psychiatric illness. In this situation, there are two basic principles which have direct therapeutic implications for the management of marital problems.

The first is that problems that arise early in the marriage are frequently related to unfulfilled expectations. Most people enter this contract hoping that the marriage will develop in a certain fashion and expect something wonderful to happen. Often these expectations are a romanticized view of what life together will be like. They may dream about all the good things and forget that the trash has to be taken out, the dishes have to be washed, and the bills have to be paid. Exaggerated expectations may be confronted by reality shortly after the honeymoon. This will be experienced as disappointment or deprivation. The husband or wife, or both, may feel cheated, as if the other person had lied; and there is a continuing spiral of recriminations, resentment, and bitterness that commonly leads toward divorce.

The second general type of problem is a differential rate of maturation. This usually appears after the couple has been married for a few years. People usually get married at a time when they suit one another's emotional needs and their personalities complement one another. After marriage, one or the other may move ahead in terms of maturity. For example, if the husband is the breadwinner, he enters the business world, meets people, and takes on responsibility. He has to develop poise to conduct his sales meetings or to interact with his associates. The demands of his work stimulate him to a more rapid maturation than his wife who might be at home or with her mother, remaining in an adolescent or even childish stage. It also happens the other way around. The husband may be working at a job, but still continuing his own adolescent activities. He may spend considerable time with "the boys" playing ball or bowling, while his wife takes over major family responsibilities such as paying bills, balancing the checkbook, taking care of the children, and solving family problems. She may be the one stimulated to mature more rapidly. After a while, this maturational difference may develop into an incompatibility which was not present at the time of marriage.

The fantasies and expectations attached to marriage are usually not mentioned spontaneously. They must be inquired about gently, with an awareness that they tend to be deeply personal and are often associated with painful disappointment. As in most psychotherapeutic efforts, it is useful to obtain detailed descriptions of the expectations. This enables the patient to communicate his or her own unique qualities and interests, and it gives the interviewer a clearer image with which to work.

Where applicable, the family physician tries to demonstrate how various aspects of the marital problem have resulted from unfulfilled expectations. Next, the physician and the couple try to discover why they have been unfulfilled. Was the patient unaware of the fantasy or its implications? Were these wishes not clearly or meaningfully communicated to the spouse? Were some of the wishes unrealistic?

The basic strategy is to determine what was desired, what is missing, and why it is missing. As the reasons for lack of fulfillment are discovered, remedies can sometimes be found. When one member understands his or her own inner wishes and those of the partner, there is often a willingness to give something desirable if the partner is willing to reciprocate. In some instances, the physician helps a person recognize that more has been expected than the spouse could humanly provide.

The problem of differential rates of maturation is more complex, but the basic approach is similar. In addition to a detailed exploration of marital expectations, it is usually necessary to obtain more information about occupational ambitions, personal goals, newly-developed interests, and attitudes toward children. It is necessary to ascertain how the couple was similar at the time of marriage and how they have become different.

It is then important to discover how this happened and what interests the couple continue to share. Ways must be sought to prevent the differences from undermining shared interests. In fact, it is often possible to help a couple enhance their mutual satisfaction by using some of their differences as advantages.

EMOTIONAL PROBLEMS THAT ACCOMPANY DEATH

The example to be discussed here is the reaction associated with the loss of a loved one and the grieving process that follows. Beginning with Eric Lindemann's classic article in 1944,[1] there have emerged in the psychiatric literature descriptions of a definite syndrome associated with ordinary grief.[2-7] Considerable experience with the problem of grief has led to the development of some basic principles of management. This information has filtered from psychiatry to family medicine with varying success. Every physician who deals with death, particularly the family physician to whom the bereaved family frequently turns for help, will be more effective in alleviating a patient's grief and preventing a pathologic reaction if he or she has a working knowledge of these principles.

The first reaction to the loss of a significant person is usually one of numb disbelief. The bereaved is unable to accept emotionally the reality and finality of the separation. It is in this shock-like state that all the details of the funeral and burial are carried out. This state of confusion between intellectual recognition of the loss and its emotional denial is enhanced as family and friends crowd about. Some time after the burial, the true impact of the loss begins to be felt. Intense pain sets in and great waves of emotion overcome the bereaved. Somatic symptoms develop, often including tightness in the throat, shortness of breath, or an empty feeling in the stomach. These waves of discomfort are precipitated by anything reminiscent of the deceased. The widow or widower may not be able to sleep at night and may complain of fatigue, exhaustion, and loss of appetite. The physician is consulted because of these physical complaints; the patient does not usually complain of grieving.

There is a considerable amount of evidence to suggest that the bereaved should be encouraged to express painful feelings openly. The most effective way for the physician to encourage the patient to express these feelings is to center the discussion around the deceased. One might stimulate a detailed recounting of a particular situation or event just prior to death.

Many patients will simply say, "Oh, Doctor, I'm so unhappy," or "Doctor, life simply is not the same." By talking in these general terms, the patient is protected from experiencing the pain that would result from a detailed description of a particular event or situation involving the deceased. Affects tend to be associated with specific experiences. The physician must direct the conversation by saying something like this: "Tell me about that birthday celebration. Where did you go? What did you wear? What did your spouse wear? What did you have for dinner?" One should encourage the bereaved to talk about the relationship with the deceased until the words flow without inhibition and carry with them a full expression of emotion.

The mental effort required to face the loss has become known as the work of grieving. As the grief work is accomplished, some noticeable lifting of the mood and lessening of somatic complaints usually occurs in 6 to 12 weeks. The average grief reaction comes to a reasonable conclusion in 6 to 12 months. In a minority of cases, dramatic improvements may occur sooner and be lasting.

In addition to encouraging the bereaved person to vocalize painful feelings, the physician should have some knowledge of the psychodynamics of grief. A major factor in grief is an acute separation anxiety. This is derived from the helplessness encountered by all infants when they cannot obtain a needed response by a parent. The infant's existence literally is dependent on the care of the parents. The adult perceives the separation from a significant other as a threat and, at some level, feels helpless. The bereaved person is alone, with no one to perform the many functions that the lost spouse once served.

The second major consideration is really another form of anxiety-guilt. There are ambivalent feelings in any significant relationship. Any hostile thoughts that were once directed against the deceased may be unconsciously believed to be responsible for the death. In addition, the bereaved may regret that some small thing he had meant to do for the deceased had not been done.

The third major dynamic element is hostility. One can be confident that in most cases of grief there are repressed feelings of desertion and abandonment. On an intellectual level, these feelings are irrational and unacceptable to the patient. The deceased did not choose to die, and it would be irreverent to be angry at the dead. Nevertheless, although the bereaved is usually not aware of them, the feelings are present on an emotional level.

The physician can enhance the healing process by anticipating that the bereaved may be containing anxiety, grief, and hostility, and by directing the discussion in a fashion that will help uncover these painful emotions. Once the patient is able to express anxiety, the physician can frequently offer reassurance that the fears are not realistic. The physician is able to aid the patient in making important decisions by helping to examine alternative options. In addition, time itself will usually prove to the bereaved that he or she is not as helpless as first imagined. The physician can support the bereaved while this is being learned.

Feelings of guilt and hostility are especially difficult to uncover. Psychiatrists have learned that these repressed feelings are frequently responsible for the development of a pathologic grief reaction. A grief reaction is considered pathologic if it is either very intense, resulting in severe or complete incapacity, or is unusually prolonged. Pathologic grief reactions may be manifested by serious and lasting psychiatric symptoms. These may include a marked depression with suicidal tendencies or regression to primitive defense mechanisms such as delusional projection, massive denial, schizoid fantasy, or outright psychosis. The patient might become completely withdrawn or exhibit immature behavior. A pathologic grief reaction once established is best managed by consulting a psychiatrist. This chapter, written for the family physician, focuses only on ordinary grief. For a discussion of pathologic grief, we refer the reader to Chapter 12 of John Nemiah's *Foundations of Psychopathology*.[8]

By gently probing and prodding, the physician may be successful in encouraging the bereaved to express overt anger toward the deceased. The tendency of the inexperienced may be to react with shock or disapproval, but this would only serve to suppress the anger further and to increase the guilt. The knowledgeable physician will help the patient by understanding and accepting this hostility as a normal element of the dynamics of grief. Furthermore, the explicit reassurance that this hostility is a normal and natural reaction to separation will help alleviate the guilt experienced by the widowed as these feelings surface. Unverbalized anger is often directed against the self, sometimes leading to depression or even to suicide.

PERSONALITY DISORDER

The one personality disorder that will be discussed in detail is the female hysterical personality disorder. The hysterical personality disorder is not yet clearly defined by psychiatry. The analytic school stresses a fixation at the Oedipal phase of psychosocial development. Others[9, 10] base this diagnosis on a constellation of behavioral traits. Furthermore, the personality disorder must be differentiated from the hysterical neurosis or classical hysterical conversion reaction. Some physicians imprecisely use the term hysterical overlay as a label for those patients who appear to be exaggerating symptoms.

Traditionally, the hysterical personality has been considered an exclusively female disorder. The recent trend to base the diagnosis on observable behavior has led to the recognition that this constellation of traits can be seen in men. Luisada[11] has reviewed a series of males with diagnosis of hysterical personality. In this chapter, the term female hysterical personality disorder is used to avoid being sexist and to underscore that we are discussing one specific aspect of a more general problem.

The female with a hysterical personality disorder can be a problem patient in family practice. If such a patient can be recognized, and the physician can devise a strategy for managing the interpersonal problems that frequently arise between patient, physician, and paramedic staff, excessive and counterproductive feelings of anger and frustration may be avoided. Furthermore, successfully helping such a patient learn to interact with others in a more appropriate fashion by engendering a mature and stable doctor-patient relationship can be rewarding for the physician, as well as for all others concerned.

Roger Peele and Stella Rubin[12] offer four general goals in the management of female hysterical personalities in a medical setting: (1) shift the patient's emphasis on control of others to control of self; (2) help her develop appropriate ways of communicating her need; (3) avoid iatrogenic drug abuse; and (4) reduce dependency to an acceptable level. The following discussion offers some concrete suggestions to the family physician for achieving these goals.

Increase Self-Control

To help the patient learn self-control, the physician must provide a model of self-control. As closeness develops in the doctor-patient relationship, the patient may feel uncomfortable and try to provoke the doctor into rejecting her. The provocations may well produce intense anger. The physician must understand the origins of this anger and remain willing to maintain a neutral stance.

At a time of confrontation, the doctor might try to interpret this process to the patient. When the physician recognizes that the patient is trying to arouse emotion, the patient can be invited to examine the interaction. The physician can say, for example, "It might be well for us to look at what is happening here," or "Let's try to understand what's going on," or "Perhaps we can figure out what this might lead to." The main idea is to present an attitude of observation in which both patient and clinician cooperate. This sort of cooperative effort is known in psychiatry as the therapeutic alliance. When the patient's cooperation has been enlisted—if only momentarily—the physician can try to translate inappropriate behavior into a verbal communication. The clinician might ask, "What did you imagine would be my reaction when you did what you just did?" or "What did you wish I would feel, do, or say?" or "What did you fear I might feel, do, or say?"

The basic strategy is to add some distance, objectivity, and perspective to the patient's intense emotional experience. As the observational process is emphasized, the patient comes to recognize that manipulation, threats, and other histrionic behaviors serve as a form of extraverbal communication. The clinician can then encourage the patient to communicate by talking rather than by acting. This change will take time. A lifelong pattern of adaptation is not easily relinquished. The clinician must help the patient to see that talking is preferable and not unduly painful. At the same time, it must be demonstrated that impulsive action is often damaging, self-defeating, irreversible, dishonorable, and contrary to the patient's ideals. The knowledgeable physician who is successful in this effort may demonstrate for the first time to the patient that she can participate in a nonthreatening relationship.

Improve Communications

The practitioner can help the patient develop appropriate ways for her to communicate needs by offering an example of clear and accurate communication. The physician should be explicit and clearly define the rules that the patient is expected to abide by in their relationship and in dealing with office staff. It is especially helpful if the patient agrees explicitly to these rules.

As an expression of her wish for intimacy, the hysterical patient will usually try to obtain more information about the personal life of the physician than is appropriate. The physician must set limits for the amount of personal information that can be comfortably shared with the patient. It is important to stress that the physician must maintain professional objectivity for the patient's sake, rather than for self-interest. Often, even calm, tactful, and reasonable refusals will be experienced as rejections, with the emergence of intense pain and anger.

The egocentric nature of the patient's personality produces a great thirst for attention. The physician is tempted to give this attention by listening to her often fascinating stories. This type of attention is counterproductive and encourages the patient to continue her inappropriate behavior. She may feel compelled to get involved in some untoward event between visits so that she has some material to give the physician. If this pattern develops, the physician might discourage her descriptions of bizarre behavior and encourage her to discuss the feelings that preceded this activity. The doctor can help the patient develop ways for communicating verbally, rather than through inappropriate behavior or suicidal gestures.

The female with a hysterical personality disorder may interact manipulatively with the office staff. The manipulative patient attempts to evoke emotions or to provoke responses in a purposeful way. Usually the patient is not conscious of that purpose, although it is often obvious to the victim and others. If the physician and staff understand that this behavior is part of the emotional disorder, a manipulation might not evoke the usual degree of anger. It is helpful for the physician to discuss the patient's behavior with the staff and encourage them to maintain a mature, neutral stance in their encounters with the patient. As previously described, the physician might initiate an open discussion with the patient of what she was trying to accomplish with this inappropriate behavior. This must be done in a nonthreatening and nonconfronting way, always emphasizing and encouraging the therapeutic alliance. The goal is to have the patient learn how to translate her behavior into more appropriate verbal communication with those about her.

It is sometimes highly productive to ask the patient how she feels when she talks to the physician. How does she imagine the physician's reaction? What does she wish or fear that the physician's attitude might be?

If there is a significant male in the patient's life, the doctor might encourage her to communicate with him in a more meaningful fashion. This intervention should take into account the anxiety that greater meaningfulness might evoke. If she can share her inner feelings with that person, she may be more successful in controlling her behavior. If the family physician also provides care for this significant male (e.g., boyfriend, husband), he might spend some time explaining to him why the patient has such an intense thirst for proof that she is loved, why she is uncomfortable with intimacy, and why she appears so dependent on him. This information may help as they try to improve their relationship. The physician should be careful not to breach the patient's confidentiality by first obtaining her informed permission to talk with the significant male. Joint conferences with the patient and her male companion can be helpful.

Avoid Iatrogenic Drug Abuse

A very simple, but important, principle is that the physician should consistently and affirmatively avoid iatrogenic drug abuse. The patient may offer varied and multiple somatic complaints. These symptoms often are presented in an exaggerated and dramatic manner. Dismissing the patient by writing a prescription can be another form of rejection. Multiple visits and multiple prescriptions expose the patient to the hazards of adverse drug reactions.

Patients with hysterical personality disorders have been shown to be susceptible to drug and alcohol addiction. Rather than freely using seda-tives and tranquilizers having the potential for addiction, we recommend that the physician reserve the benzodiazepines for severe anxiety, and the tricyclics for marked depression. Use of any medication should be made with exceptional caution and parsimony.

Reduce Dependency

The physician may help the patient reduce dependency on people in general by not allowing her to become too dependent on the physician. This can be accomplished most effectively through interpretation of the process. "How do you feel when you ask me to decide (do, prevent, advise) something for you?" "How do you feel when I do it?" "How do you feel when I don't?" The clinician can encourage the patient to take an active role in her own medical care. If the physician becomes involved in formal counseling, the temptation to give advice should be avoided. The physician must avoid offering reassurance—as contrasted with hope —about the future. It is most effective to encourage the patient to ex-amine her own behavior or to examine alternative possibilities, and then reach her own conclusions. When dealing with issues of dependency, the patient can assume responsibility. She should receive recognition for even minor changes in behavior that might help foster her sense of indepen-dence.

CONCLUSION

The common problems listed in Table 9-1 are frequently encountered in family medicine. The family physician must be able to recognize these problems and be prepared to manage them. These problems may be man-aged by the physician alone or in collaboration with a mental health pro-fessional. In either instance, the physician requires interviewing skills to uncover information and formulate the nature of the patient's problem. This must be accomplished before a course of management, with or with-out the help of others, can be outlined.

The current emphasis on behavioral science and psychiatry in family practice residency programs will hopefully produce a new generation of family physicians better prepared to recognize the psychosocial prob-lems that underlie many patient complaints. The interested and well-prepared physician of the future should also be able to contribute greatly to the recognition and management of these conditions.

REFERENCES

1. Lindemann E: Symptomatology and management of acute grief. Am J Psychiatry 101:141, 1944
2. Bornstein PE, Clayton PJ, Halikas JA, et al: The depression of widowhood after thirteen months. Br J Psychiatry 122:561, 1973
3. Clayton PJ, Halikas JA, Maurice WL: The bereavement of the widowed. Dis Nerv Syst 32:597, 1971
4. Clayton PJ, Halikas JA, Maurice WL: The depression of widowhood. Br J Psychiatry 120:71, 1972
5. Clayton PJ: Mortality and morbidity in the first year of widowhood. Arch Gen Psychiatry 30:747, 1974
6. Clayton PJ, Herjanis M, Murphy GE, et al: Mourning and depression: Their similarities and differences. Can Psychiatr Assoc J 19:309, 1974
7. Messsner E, Schmidt D: Videotape in the training of medical students in psychiatric aspects of family medicine. Int J Psychiatry Med 5:269, 1974
8. Nemiah JC: *Foundations of Psychopathology*. New York: Oxford University Press, 1961, Chaps. 10, 12
9. Alarcon RD: Hysteria and hysterical personality: How come one without the other? Psychoanal 47:258, 1973
10. American Psychiatric Association: *Diagnostic and Statistical Manual of Mental Disorders*, 3rd ed. Washington, DC: American Psychiatric Association, 1968
11. Luisada PV, Peele R, Pittard EA: The hysterical personality in men. Am J Psychiatry 131:518, 1974
12. Peele R, Rubin, SI: The hysterical personality: Identifying and managing one of the problem patients of medical practice. South Med J 67:679, 1974

CHAPTER 10

ASSESSMENT OF FAMILY FUNCTION

GABRIEL SMILKSTEIN

INTRODUCTION

Assessment and management of family function as it has been practiced in the tradition of the general and family physician is now under study in many academic departments of family medicine. The aim of these studies is to develop a body of knowledge that can be shared with students, resident physicians, and practitioners, so that they may approach the psychosocial issues of family dysfunction as competently as biomedical problems.

Most patient-physician encounters in family practice relate to the problems of the individual patient; however, physicians know that illness produces some degree of dysfunction in the family. It has also been recognized that when the family unit is stressed, members will undergo some measure of psychophysiological impairment.[1, 2]

Family crises, past and present, are stressful life events that have produced disequilibrium or dysfunction among family members or between the family and community. As discussed in Chapter 2, the degree to which a crisis alters the family function depends upon its impact. The factors that influence the impact of crisis are (1) the level of family function at the onset of the crisis; (2) the significance of the crisis to the family; and (3) the resources available to the family.

If the family is rich in resources, the physician may not be called for assistance. However, in times of crises of major impact, such as a serious illness, divorce, death, or juvenile delinquency, a resource-poor family may become dysfunctional. At such times family members require support and guidance from a physician who is knowledgeable about family function, the impact of the crisis, and appropriate therapies.

DEFINITION OF FAMILY FUNCTION

Murdock, a sociologist who studied comparative family function in various cultures, described the universal family functions as (1) reproduction; (2) sexual role definition; (3) economic cooperation; and (4) socialization of offspring.[3] As with many definitions of family, Murdock's fulfills the needs of the field of study from which it was derived. Tables 10-1 and 10-2 illustrate how definitions of family may vary according to the adapted conceptual framework. New definitions of family in current use suggest that family structure and function should be determined by the individuals who comprise the family.[5] For example, two persons of the same sex, unrelated genetically or legally, may share intellectual, sexual, and emotional needs and gratifications, a dwelling place, clothing and food, yet carry out independent and unrelated reproductive functions. These individuals may determine the form and function which they desire their family to have, uninfluenced by social norms for struc-

TABLE 10-1.   Structural Definitions of Family*

Family of Orientation:	The nuclear family in which a person has had the status of child.[4]
Family of Procreation:	The nuclear family in which a person has or had the status of parent.[4]
Extended Family:	Any grouping whose members are related by descent, marriage, or adoption; broader than the nuclear family.[4]
Joint Family:	Various groups of nuclear families, usually related biologically, who share property rights.[4]
Polygamous Family:	Two or more nuclear families affiliated by plural marriage (e.g., one man, two women, and progeny).[4]

* Source: Baumer J, Smilkstein G: *Family: A Definition for Family Physicians.*[5]

TABLE 10-2. Anthropological, Sociological, and Psychological Definitions of Family*

Institutional Framework:	Focuses on the origin and evolution of the family institution with comparisons over space and time of its relationships to different societies and cultures.[6]
Structural/Functional Framework:	Defines family by the relationships of its members to each other and existing social systems. Concentrates on how family systems are organized and operate.[7]
Interactional Framework:	Conceives of the family as a "unity of interacting personalities," "a living, changing, growing thing" in which family member interactions include role playing, status relations, and socialization processes.[8]
Situational Framework:	Focuses on the family as a social situation; "a unified set of stimuli external to the family members" capable of affecting the individual's behavior within the family and capable of being affected by other groups as well.[9]
Developmental Framework:	Views the family as the recognizable social institution consisting of interacting personalities, changing through time. It focuses attention on the longitudinal career of the family and its life-cycle.[10]

* Source: Baumer J, Smilkstein G: *Family: A Definition for Family Physicians.*[5]

ture and function. Some contemporary definitions reflecting the influence of the individual in establishing family structure and function are listed in Table 10-3.

The family physician who is sought by the patient to reestablish family equilibrium requires a working definition of family function highlighting the patient-family relationship. Richardson, who made the first definitive American contribution by a physician to the literature on family function, claimed that the interactional relationship among family members should be the focus of concern for the family physician.[16] As a unit for study and treatment, the family was viewed as a homeostatic system; change in one part could produce a psychophysiological reaction in another. This generalization suggested a rationale for the study of the family as a dynamic unit ever reacting to stressful life events.

Since family function may be highly unstable and variable, the following definition is offered to physicians as a conceptual framework for understanding the structure and function of families under their care:

TABLE 10-3. Family Definitions Dependent Upon Roles of Members*

Family:	Any socially sanctioned relationship between nonsanguinely related, cohabiting adults of opposite sex which satisfies mutual, symmetrical or complementary felt needs.[11]
Family:	Any cohabiting domestic relationship which is or has been sexually consequential; i.e., resulting in gratification of partners or in reproduction.[12]
Cohabitation:	A heterosexual couple without a legal contract who consistently share a living facility.[13]
Commune:	A relationship of individuals who agree to make life commitments as members of one particular group rather than many different groups.[14]
Group Marriage:	A multilateral marriage in which each of three or more people consider themselves to have a primary relationship with at least two other individuals in the group.[15]

* Source: Baumer J, Smilkstein G: *Family: A Definition for Family Physicians.*[5]

The family is a psychosocial system consisting of the patient and one or more persons—children and/or adults—in which there is a commitment to nurture each other.[17]

In this definition, the structure is defined as the patient and one or more persons. Clarification of the relationships in a family may be obtained by noting the family members such as husband-wife-child, grandmother-grandchild, lover-lover. Family physicians may also need to determine genetic relationships accurately in order to evaluate problems related to inherited disease, legal relationships, or to establish responsibility for care. Therefore, a particular family structure, as elaborated in a family tree,[18] may be helpful in assessing certain family problems.

Understanding the use of the word nurture is central to an understanding of family function. In the above definition of family, nurture means to sustain life, to promote the development of the emotional, intellectual, and physical growth of each family member. This ideal is achieved through a number of activities that have been identified by various authors as critical components of family function.

Sussmann claims that the components of family function that most influence the interactional response of family members are (1) socialization of children; (2) enhancement of competence in coping; (3) assistance in utilization of community resources; (4) encouragement in identity development; and (5) providing for affectional response.[19]

Pratt, who studies family function and health behavior, labeled as "energized" the family that mastered the following five areas of function:

(1) maintained varied and regular family interaction with each other; (2) established ties to the broader community through the active participation of members in extra-familial social systems; (3) encouraged autonomy of family members; (4) creatively problem-solved through the use of quality family resources; and (5) adjusted to role changes within the family.[20] The latter was considered of some importance by Spiegel, who held that role definition and complementarity were of major importance in maintaining interactional equilibrium in a family.[21]

The Family APGAR, a family function questionnaire to be later discussed in this chapter, utilizes five components of family function described in Table 10-4.[22] The conceptual basis for the Family APGAR is that the well-being of a family is predicated on the success with which family members achieve adaptation (coping), partnership (role complementarity), growth (identity development), affection (emotional understanding), and resolve (commitment to share). Disequilibrium or functional impairment of a family is pathologically manifested by one or more of these components.

EVALUATION OF FAMILY FUNCTION

When a family member reports the history of a crisis to a physician, the general status of this family's function can usually be discovered. Considerable information about family function may be obtained when the patient describes how family members communicate, eat, sleep, and carry out home, school, and job responsibilities.[23] Depression may also be a sign of failure to cope. Therefore, the patient reporting a family crisis

TABLE 10-4. The Five Components of Family Function (Family APGAR)*

1. **Adaptation:** the utilization of intra- and extra-familial resources for problem-solving in times of crisis.
2. **Partnership:** the sharing of decision-making and nurturing responsibilities by family members.
3. **Growth:** the physical and emotional maturation and self-fulfillment that is achieved by family members through mutual support and guidance.
4. **Affection:** the caring or loving relationship that exists among family members.
5. **Resolve:** the commitment to devote time to other members of the family for physical and emotional nurturing; involving a decision to share wealth and space.

* Smilkstein G: *The Family in Crisis.*[22]

(especially one of abandonment) should be questioned regarding symptoms of depression (e.g., suicide, isolation, constipation, early morning wakening, and loss of appetite). Evidence of dysfunction in any of these areas should alert the physician to the need to evaluate family function in greater depth.

The problem that has faced the physician wishing to gain more complete information on family function is the dearth of pragmatic evaluation instruments. Many questionnaires and procedures have been devised to establish the state of the family functional integrity; however, because of their complexity, length, or limited focus[24, 25] they fail to meet the needs of the practicing physician. A number of questionnaires center on the marital relationship in general[26-29] or on particular aspects of the husband-wife relationship: communication,[30, 31] decisionmaking,[32] or parental roles.[33, 34] Others assess family function more broadly, from the perspective of children[35, 36] or adults.[37, 38] Many of these instruments have been used in research protocols and as such are inappropriate for use by the practicing physician.[37-41]

In 1973, Pless and Satterwhite introduced a Family Function Index (FFI) that was developed as a "simple, easily-administered test to reflect the dynamics of family interaction."[25, 42] The FFI consists of 15 questions and requires about 15 minutes to administer. It estimates family function by evaluating areas of nuclear family interaction such as marital satisfaction, frequency of disagreement, communication, problem-solving, and feelings of happiness and closeness. The reliability of the FFI was established by comparing index scores with ratings of the same families by experienced case workers. The FFI has been used to study the nuclear families of children with chronic physical disorders, and its authors claim to identify accurately which chronically ill children are likely to experience secondary psychological difficulties.

The Family APGAR, a questionnaire that features five closed-ended questions, was developed as a multi-dimensional measure of global family function.[17] It was designed to be short, easy to score, and suitable for diverse family constellations, in addition to traditional nuclear families. The APGAR acronym has been applied since physicians are familiar with the Apgar[43] evaluation of the newborn and are likely to remember a similar format that scores the functional status of a family.

The questions in the Family APGAR are designed to permit qualitative measurement of the family member's satisfaction with each of the five basic components of family function. Table 10-5 lists the functional components of the Family APGAR and indicates the qualitative data that may be obtained.

Data from the family function evaluation will not only give the physician an estimate of the family's coping capabilities, but may also serve

TABLE 10-5.   Family APGAR Questionnaire*

	Almost always	Some of the time	Hardly ever
I am satisfied that I can turn to my family when something is troubling me.	⎯⎯	⎯⎯	⎯⎯
I am satisfied with the way my family talks over things with me and shares problems with me.	⎯⎯	⎯⎯	⎯⎯
I am satisfied that my family accepts and supports my wishes to take on new activities or directions.	⎯⎯	⎯⎯	⎯⎯
I am satisfied with the way my family expresses affection and responds to my emotions, such as anger, sorrow, and love.	⎯⎯	⎯⎯	⎯⎯
I am satisfied with the way my family and I share time together.	⎯⎯	⎯⎯	⎯⎯

Scoring: The patient checks one of three choices which are scored as follows: "Almost always" (2 points), "Some of the time" (1 point), or "Hardly ever" (0). The scores for each of the five questions are then totaled. A score of 7 to 10 suggests a highly functional family. A score of 4 to 6 suggests a moderately dysfunctional family. A score of 0 to 3 suggests a severely dysfunctional family.

* Adapted from Smilkstein G: *The Family APGAR: A Proposal for a Family Function Test and Its Use by Physicians.*[17]

as a lead in initiating a discussion. For example, if the patient scores zero on the question, "I am satisfied with the way my family and I share time together," the physician can use an open-ended question such as "I see that you have a problem with the amout of time that your family spends together. Tell me about it." In this manner, the questionnaire helps the physician to quickly focus on the critical problems of the family in trouble.

The validity of the Family APGAR was established by administering the questionnaire to two samples, believed to have relatively high and relatively low family function respectively.[44] High function was attributed to married graduate students at a university housing project, and low scores to patients in a mental health clinic. Additionally, scores obtained on the Family APGAR were compared with scores on a measure of family function of established validity and reliability (Pless and Satterwhite's Family Function Index),[25, 42] and evaluations of family function by clinical therapists. As hypothesized, there was a significant difference between the Family APGAR scores of the clinic patients and the married graduate students. Out of a possible total score of 10, the mean score was 8.24 for the married graduate students and 5.89 for the clinic patients.

Thirty-three respondents in the married graduate student group completed both the Family APGAR and the Pless-Satterwhite questionnaire. There was a strong correlation of .80 between the Family APGAR score and the Pless-Satterwhite score. A moderately high correlation of .64 between the Family APGAR score and the therapists' family evaluation score was attained for the clinic group.

CLINICAL APPLICATIONS OF THE FAMILY APGAR

Three situations have been identified in which the physician may need information on the functional state of the patient's family.

1. Family function data may be needed when a new patient is introduced into a physician's practice. There is merit in seeing that family as a unit on at least one occasion;[45] such an encounter allows the physician to gain some insight into family interaction. While the interview process does not usually allow the physician time to gain an adequate view of the status of family function, giving the Family APGAR questionnaire to the whole family permits the physician to establish a baseline view of family function. Just as the Pediatric Apgar uses 1- and 5-minute evaluations to judge the progress of a newborn infant, the family physician may wish to administer the Family APGAR at the first visit and repeat it at intervals to judge the changes in a family's functional status.

2. Functional information is needed when the family will be involved in the patient's care. All illnesses and injuries represent some measure of stress to the family.[46] Thus, in the case of a patient with coronary artery disease, information on family function would assist in ascertaining the patient's ability to return home as a passive convalescent. A high Family APGAR score would suggest that the family can adapt to the crisis of the patient's illness and role change. A low score would warn the physician that the home environment could be stressful to the coronary patient; the physician might then wish to take a closer look at family member interaction before sending the patient home.

3. Family function information is essential when the physician is involved in managing a family in trouble. When a family crisis is reported to the physician, it indicates that the family's resources are inadequate to cope with a problem. In this situation the Family APGAR questionnaire can highlight specific areas of weakness that interfere with

family members' ability to communicate or identify resources. Family members' responses also provide leads in initiating a discussion, as previously illustrated.

The following case history serves to demonstrate the use of the Family APGAR during a crisis episode:

Mrs. Jackson, a 39-year-old black, married, junior-college educator, was hospitalized with generalized urticaria. This rash had appeared in a milder form during the spring 2 years prior to her admission, and was easily controlled with antihistamines and steroids. However, on this occasion it had resisted therapy. Hospitalization was advised to control the pruritis and attempt to identify the etiology of the urticaria.

Biomedical studies were nonproductive. A diagnosis of idiopathic urticaria and atopic dermatitis was established. An investigation of Mrs. Jackson's psychosocial background yielded a history of numerous crises. Directly related to previous episodes of generalized urticaria, there was an associated history of failure to receive an administrative appointment the patient felt she deserved. At home she was not allowed to express anger about this disappointment since her husband, a pastor with a small, struggling congregation, felt an expression of anger or disappointment inappropriate; he felt all that happened in life reflected God's will.

Family history revealed that an only son died of sickle cell anemia. The circumstances surrounding this death were unusual. The child was taken to the local emergency room with symptoms of cough and fever. He was admitted to the hospital with a diagnosis of pneumonia, and the parents were encouraged to go home. During the night the child died. A policeman called at the family's home in the morning to notify the parents of the child's death. Although the patient and her husband were upset with the way the matter had been handled, they did not complain to the authorities. The result was a prolonged grief reaction. During a later interview family residual anger was evident even after a period of 7 years had elapsed.

Mr. Jackson's inability to express feelings of anger resulted in a projection of these emotions onto his wife. For example, he was disappointed with the fact that he did not have a son to carry his name. During a counseling session he stated that "my wife is very disappointed that we don't have a son." Mrs. Jackson did not support this statement at any time.

Another area of apparent conflict related to Mrs. Jackson having a master's degree and a white collar income; her husband's education was limited to Bible college and his church barely survived financially. The disparity in education and income was not an issue for discussion in the home. The couple maintained a patriarchal household (i.e., husband/father dominated).

Aside from these stressful life events, there were a number of minor crises related to the husband's arthritic knee and sickle cell anemia in the youngest daughter. The daughter's problem resulted in two to three yearly hospitalizations.

During Mrs. Jackson's hospitalization, evidence of psychosocial crises suggested the value of a family function study. The Family APGAR scores for this family were:

Mrs. Jackson	8
Mr. Jackson	8
Daughter (age 18)	9
Daughter (age 16)	9
Daughter (age 12)	9

At first glance the family appears highly functional with top level Family APGAR scores. Yet, an analysis of the questionnaires and a review of the family's psychosocial history revealed that the family had a high level of pathology that Minuchin would label as "enmeshment".[46] This suggests a family where the involvement of members in each other's lives results in a major yielding of individual autonomy. There was a significant subsystem of husband-wife and mother-children. These subsystems were in conflict with each other and resulted in the isolation of the husband/father, children, and wife/mother. To maintain equilibrium, Mrs. Jackson had to give in to the requests of her husband who wished to maintain power, and give up her urban views of assertiveness and participation in problem-solving.

The Family APGAR responses submitted by this family offered support for the enmeshment diagnosis and allowed the family physician who managed the counseling sessions to identify primary problem areas. Mr. Jackson scored low on expression of feelings, as well as time spent with family. He added these comments: (1) "I don't show anger to any member of my family" and (2) "I am content, but not satisfied."

Mrs. Jackson scored low on partnership (satisfaction with her husband's discussion of items of common interest), and growth (satisfaction that husband is willing to take on new activities). The daughters all scored low on growth (satisfaction with parents, particularly Mr. Jackson's, willingness to take on new activities).

The outcome of the counseling session was an improved dialogue in the family regarding the critical issues described above. Mr. Jackson was able to discuss his anger and sense of isolation. The women in the family accepted their reponsibility to help Mr. Jackson maintain his congregation, balanced with some recognition of their own needs. Mrs. Jackson did not manifest any urticarial reaction during the 2 months of counseling.

The Family APGAR scores for the Jackson family demonstrate the importance of placing laboratory results in context with the data base obtained during an interview. Values of 7–10 on the Family APGAR usually suggest a functional family; however, in families such as the Jacksons, a high score may reflect family dysfunction due to pathologic enmeshment that members have in each others' lives. In these families, overprotection is manifested by denial or suppression of problems, resulting in a fantasized or idealized family.

CONCLUSIONS

Physicians should recognize that the goal of family function assessment is to assist in the recognition of family problems. This does not mean that all families will be salvageable. There will be times when the process of diagnosis, therapy, and consultation fail and the family must consider the options of separation or divorce. However, the physician who can effectively identify psychosocial family problems is more likely to help a family resolve its problems.

REFERENCES

1. Haley J: Whither family therapy? Fam Process 1:69–100, 1962
2. Caplan G: *Principles of Preventive Psychiatry.* New York: Bennie Books, Inc., 1964, p. 40
3. Murdock GP: "The Universality of the Nuclear Family." In Bell NW, Vogel EF eds: *A Modern Introduction to the Family,* rev. ed. New York: The Free Press, 1968, pp. 37–47
4. Bell NW and Vogel EF: "Toward a Framework for Functional Analysis of Family Behavior." In Bell NW, Vogel EF eds: *A Modern Introduction to the Family,* rev. ed. New York: The Free Press, 1968, pp. 1–34
5. Baumer J, Smilkstein G: *Family: A Definition for Family Physicians.* University of California at Davis: Department of Family Practice, (unpublished Family Practice Fellowship paper, 1975)
6. Goode WJ: *World Revolution and Family Patterns.* New York: The Free Press, 1970, pp. 366–380
7. Bell NW and Vogel EF eds: *A Modern Introduction to the Family,* rev. ed. New York: The Free Press, 1968, pp. 7–34
8. Schaneveldt JD: "The Interactional Framework in the Study of the Family." In Nye IF, Berrardo FM eds: *Emerging Conceptual Frameworks in Family Analysis.* New York: Macmillan Company, 1966, pp. 92–129
9. Bossard JHS, Ball ES: *Family Situations.* Philadelphia: University of Pennsylvania Press, 1943, pp. 37–56
10. Hill R, Rodgers RH: "The Developmental Approach." In Christensen HT ed: *Handbook of Marriage and the Family.* Chicago: Rand McNally and Company, 1964, pp. 171–211
11. Ball DW: The family as a sociological problem: Conceptualization of the taken-for-granted as a prologue to social problems analysis. Soc Prob 19:67–88, 1972
12. Spiro ME: Is the family universal? Amer Anthro 56:839–846, 1954
13. Clatworthy NM: "Living Together." In Glazer-Malkin H ed: *Old Family/New Family.* New York: D. Van Nostrand Company, 1973, pp. 67–89
14. Ramey JW: "Emerging Patterns of Innovative Marriage." In Sussman M ed: *Nontraditional Family Forms in the 1970s.* Minneapolis: National Council on Family Relations, 1972, pp. 57–64
15. Constantine L, Constantine JM: "Dissolution of Marriage in a Nonconventional Context." In Sussman M ed: *Nontraditional Family Forms in the 1970s.* Minneapolis: National Council on Family Relations, 1972, pp. 89–94
16. Richardson HR: *Patients Have Families.* Cambridge, Mass: Commonwealth Fund, Harvard University Press, 1948, pp. 48–76
17. Smilkstein G: The family APGAR: A proposal for a family function test and its use by physicians. J Fam Prac 6:1231–1239, 1978

18. Rakel RE: *Principles of Family Medicine.* Philadelphia: W. B. Saunders Company, 1977, pp. 478–489
19. Sussman MB: "Family Systems in the 1970s: Analysis, Policies and Programs." In Hymovich DP, Barnard MM eds: *Family Health Care.* New York: McGraw-Hill, 1973, p. 25
20. Pratt L: *Family Structure and Effective Health Behavior.* Boston: Houghton Mifflin Company, 1976, p. 156
21. Spiegel JP: The resolution of role conflict within the family. Psychiatry 20:1–16, 1957
22. Smilkstein G: "The Family in Crisis." In Taylor R ed: *Family Medicine: Principles and Practice.* New York: Springer-Verlag, 1978
23. Hoff LA: *People in Crisis: Understanding and Helping.* Menlo Park, California: Addison-Wesley, 1978, p. 53
24. Strauss MA: *Measurement Techniques: Abstracts of Published Instruments, 1935–1965.* Minneapolis: University of Minnesota Press, 1969
25. Pless B, Satterwhite B: A measure of family function and its application. Soc Sci Med 7:613, 1973
26. Weiss RL, Hops H, Patterson GR: "A Framework for Conceptualizing Marital Conflict, a Technology for Altering It, Some Data for Evaluating It." In Clark FW, Hamerlynck LA eds: *Critical Issues in Research and Practice: Proceedings of the Fourth Banff International Conference in Behavior Modification.* Champaign, Illinois: Research Press, 1973
27. Birchler GR, Well LJ: Discriminating interaction behaviors in happy and unhappy marriages. J Consult Clin Psychol 45:494, 1977
28. Bowerman CE: Adjustment in marriage: Overall and in specific areas. Sociol Soc Res 41:257–263, 1957
29. Buerkle JV, Badgley RF: Couple role taking: The Yale marital interaction battery. Marriage Fam Liv 21:53–58, 1959
30. Hobart CW, Klausner WJ: Some social interactional correlates of marital role disagreement and marital adjustment. Marriage Fam Liv 21:256–263, 1959
31. Karlsson G: *Adaptability and Communication in Marriage: A Swedish Predictive Study of Marital Satisfaction.* Uppsala: Almquist & Wiksells, 1951
32. Blood RO, Jr., Wolfe DM: *Husbands and Wives: The Dynamics Of Married Living.* Glencoe, Illinois: The Free Press, 1960
33. Hoffman ML: An interview method for obtaining descriptions of parent-child interaction. Merrill-Palmer Quart 4:76–83, 1957
34. Meyer MM, Tollman RS: Correspondence between attitudes and images of parental figures in TAT stories and in therapeutic interviews. J Consult Clin Psychol 19:79–82, 1955
35. Bronfenbrenner U: "Toward a Theoretical Model for the Analysis of Parent-Child Relationships in a Social Context." In Glidewell JC ed: *Parental Attitudes and Child Behavior.* Springfield, Illnois: C. C. Thomas, 1961
36. Brown AW, Morrison J, Couch GB: Influence of affectional family relationships on character development. J Abnorm Psych 42:422–29, 1947
37. Myers TR: Intra-family relationships and pupil adjustment. Teach Coll Contr Educ No. 651, 1940
38. Geismar LL, LaSorte MA, Ayres B: Measuring family disorganization. Marriage Fam Liv 24:51–56, 1962

39.   Cavan R and Ranck K: *The Family and the Depression*. Chicago: University of Chicago Press, 1938
40.   Brim OG, Jr., Fairchild RW, Borgatta EF: Relations between family problems. Marriage Fam Liv 23:219–226, 1961
41.   Arbogast RC, Scratton JM, Krich JP: The family as patient: Preliminary experience with a recorded assessment schema. J Fam Pract 7:1151–7, 1978
42.   Pless IB, Satterwhite B: "Family Function and Family Problems." In Haggerty RJ, Roughman HS, Pless IB eds: *Child Health and the Community*. New York: John Wiley and Sons, 1975
43.   Apgar V: A proposal for a new method of evaluation of the newborn infant. Curr Res in Anesth and Analges 32:260–267, 1953
44.   Good DM-J, Smilkstein G, Good BJ, Shaffer T, Arons T: The family APGAR index: A study of construct validity. J Fam Pract 8:577–582, 1979
45.   Bauman MH, Grace NT: Family process and family practice. J Fam Pract 1:24, 1974
46.   Minuchin S: *Families and Family Therapy*. Cambridge, Mass: Harvard University Press, 1974

CHAPTER 11

THE MENTAL STATUS EXAMINATION

HIRAM B. CURRY

The 25,000 psychiatrists in this country cannot meet the needs of more than twenty-million people in the United States with mental and emotional problems. The majority of these can be diagnosed and managed by family physicians and other adequately trained health care professionals. In addition, up to 75 percent of all persons consulting physicians for physical symptoms have complicating or contributing emotional and/or social problems.[1] Optimal health care requires attention of physical, emotional, and social aspects of the problem.

In some ways, the work of the family physician may be more difficult than that of a psychiatrist or psychologist. The latter often see patients who have been screened and found to have problems which require specialized psychiatric attention. However, the family physician must frequently decide if there is a problem and what care is required. Many patients do not seem able to come to their physician for an emotional problem. Perhaps they feel that such problems are a sign of weakness. At an unconscious level, the problem can then be somatized, and a visit to the physician acceptable. The challenge for the family physician is clear. It is to listen carefully to the patient, hear and understand the vague, nonspecific, and often unclassifiable complaints, tease them apart, and recognize a familiar pattern suggesting problems that are medical, emotional, mental, social, or a mixture of factors.

The family physician's ability to deal with the wide range of problems presented by patients is a test of the physician's understanding of the human condition. To be involved enough to be caring, yet distant enough to be objective is a test of the physician's stability. The patient's personality, and hostility, demands, need to manipulate, suspiciousness, seductiveness or litigious behavior can greatly color any complaint, and significantly affect the physician's ability to appraise it accurately. The physician must be aware of any negative feelings, and control or counter them.

Most medical graduates are frustrated if they cannot make a medical diagnosis quickly and easily. The experienced clinician realizes that emotional reactions to a disease may produce more symptoms and be more evident than the symptoms of the underlying disease. In these instances, an understanding of the mental and emotional status of the patient is very important if the problem is to be correctly diagnosed. In addition, emotional disturbance accompanying the illness may finally determine the response to treatment, and the time required for the patient's return to a normal pattern of living.

An important and seldom acknowledged clue to diagnosis is the physician's own feelings while with the patient; indeed, his response to the patient's feelings. An intuitive physician may feel the deep distress of the patient before the details of the situation are stated, or even if they are not available. A sensitive physician may feel his own mood slide downward as he sits and talks with the depressed patient. Unfortunately, many physicians are not sufficiently in touch with their own feelings to utilize them to advantage in the clinical situation. Many medical scientists consider such data too soft and lacking in objectivity to be useful. The sensitive, intuitive, and experienced physician can use feelings to good advantage.

ASSESSMENT OF MENTAL STATUS

Mental status evaluation is indicated in any condition where there is suffering and/or disability resulting from a thinking, feeling or behavioral disorder. Mental status evaluation is very similar to evaluation for a physical problem. There is the history, then the examination of the patient followed by special tests. The purpose of the examination is to evaluate the organ of the mind, to determine the patient's emotional state, mental capacity, and functioning status. This evaluation is more difficult than the physical examination, especially if the patient resents the procedure, is highly nervous, or is otherwise uncooperative. In these instances the examiner must use judgment and ingenuity.

The patient needing evaluation of mental status may come to the attention of the family physician in several ways:

1. The physician notes a decline during professional visits or social encounters.
2. Family member or business associate notes changes and urges evaluation.
3. The patient notes a decline in his own functioning.
4. A sudden problem erupts which may reach crisis proportions.

When a patient is acutely disturbed the following questions are useful to quickly appraise the situation:

1. Has the patient had a similar episode in the past? If the patient has had similar episodes in the past, the diagnosis and what has been a successful management program may be known by a family member. The temporal profile of every physical, mental or emotional illness is the basic and most important diagnostic feature every clinician uses. Its importance cannot be overestimated.

2. Does the patient have a known systemic disease? When a change in behavior occurs in one with a known organic disease, that disease should be considered as a primary diagnostic possibility. Certain diseases are known for their effect on the central nervous system: carcinoma of the pancreas and depression, lupus erythematosus and psychosis, metastatic carcinoma and personality change.

3. What circumstances precipitated the event? Interpretation of the circumstances that precipitate a behavioral event requires judgment on the part of the physician. An extreme event may cause most persons to respond irrationally. Our concern then is to define whether or not the event was precipitated by trivial irritations or by an irrational perception of the situation. Not only the event is important, but also its background and the nature of the precipitating factors.

4. Has the patient's mood been normal? A history of an earlier period of extreme elation may be highly useful in interpreting the significance of a prolonged period of sadness, or in diagnosing bipolar affective disease.

5. Does the patient take prescribed medications, illicit substances, or alcohol? Information regarding prescribed and illicit drugs and alcohol should be confirmed by seeing the medication containers and by second-party history. A careful drug history may provide important clues for symptoms which may have lead to the mental status examination.

6. Has the patient's behavior suggested abnormal perception of

reality? Family members may report the patient has been communicating with nonexistent people. The behavior of the schizophrenic may suggest active auditory hallucinations.

7.   Has the patient lost the ability to perform any physical or intellectual task? Before dementia can be diagnosed, a loss of previously attained intellectual ability must be proven. This requires that the level of earlier intellectual functioning be ascertained. This is best illustrated by specifying what the patient could do one year or one month earlier and what can be done now. Carefully recorded data of this type can help the physician estimate the rate of loss or the rate of recovery from a treatable disease.

A basic rule to be observed when evaluating a person with disturbed mental or emotional status is the second-party history. The patient with disturbed perception may relate to friends and associates in a quite different manner, telling a different story than is told the physician. This same clinical rule must be observed when there have been unconscious periods, periods of disorientation, seizures, or an altered state of consciousness due to alcohol or drugs.

Interviewing family members and close associates also is vital when the patient's illness has adversely affected memory or ability to observe or comprehend. Through lack of insight the patient may be unaware of the illness, even the chief complaint. Inquiry should be made about the patient's general behavior, capacity for work, personal habits, memory, and judgment. Such discussions may reveal serious problems and tensions between family members which may be contributing to the patient's emotional problems. The physician may discover that the patient's problems are symptomatic of a family illness.

Weitzel et al. have developed a mental status examination including 15 items agreed upon as being important by 28 professors of psychiatry in this country.[2] They recommended that a form be followed to ensure completeness and to favor conciseness. The following modification utilizing 14 items is recommended for the family physician. It will be obvious that these items are only a part of the basis for understanding the patient with a mental or emotional problem, just as the physical examination is only a part of the total evaluation of a physically ill patient. These items are:

1.   **Behavior during evaluation.** The examiner should note whether the patient is anxious or apathetic, interested or disinterested, passive or dramatically active, cooperative or resistant, friendly or hostile. The patient may be suspicious or manipulative. The degree of the patient's concern for the implications of the problem is of great importance. Inappropriate absence of concern (La Belle Indifference) is seen regularly in hysterical syndromes.

2. **Orientation to person, place, and time.** Does the patient know who he or she is, who the examiner is, and where the patient is? Can the patient state the time, day, month, and year? Is the patient stuporous, sleepy, dull, or alert to the surroundings? Correct orientation depends upon conscious awareness; it requires accurate perception, comprehension, and a good memory.

3. **Dress and personal habits.** Whether the patient is meticulously dressed or dirty, untidy, and unsuitably dressed may be important clues to compulsive behavior, depression, or schizophrenia. The degree and regularity of drug and alcohol usage should be described in detail.

4. **Motor behavior and speech.** The examiner should note whether the patient is withdrawn and inactive or is hyperactive and pacing, carrying out repetitive or compulsive acts. Peculiar mannerisms and unusual movements such as a tremor, chorea, athetosis, and dystonia can be important clues for an accurate diagnosis. As the evaluation proceeds and certain items are discussed, there may be a significant behavioral change. Such clues should be recorded, and it is important to note if the body language agrees with the patient's words.

Some patients will be preoccupied with particular thoughts that require motor responses. Does the patient talk endlessly about the same subject, possibly indicating recurrent ideas or an obsession? Does the patient engage in rituals to allay anxiety, or perform ridiculous acts explaining that they are required by compulsions?

The examiner must determine if the patient can communicate a particular idea successfully. Does the patient become derailed by allowing secondary or associated thoughts to displace the main idea? Is the speed and force of speech within normal limits? Do words used by the patient or movement within the room, cause the patient to change subjects, even in the middle of a sentence? This may indicate that the patient's associations are loose, as seen in schizophrenia.

5. **Memory.** It is desirable to test recent memory (the last six months) and past or remote memory (more than six months ago). Immediate recall memory is tested by having the patient remember specific items for several minutes (e.g., book, pencil, and yellow rose). After several minutes, while the patient is tested in other areas, the examiner asks for the items to be repeated. If the patient reminds the examiner that the information was not subsequently requested, it may indicate that the patient has a better memory than the examiner!

Memory testing should be done under optimal conditions if the results are to be valid. If the patient has many pressing worries competing for attention, or if there are activities and distractions in the examining room, the test should be postponed and/or moved.

Every patient is using memory as complaints and experiences are described to the physician. As a part of testing memory, one should inquire about everyday life events. This information and its orderliness and consistency can be used as an important source of data for evaluating memory. When there is doubt about accuracy then a second-party history or other documentation becomes essential.

The simplest test of memory is repeating random single-digit numbers. These should be stated in a normal voice at a rate of about one per second. Care should be taken to avoid familiar groups of numbers, for they are the memory equivalent of one item, e.g., 747 or 666. The examiner determines the number of digits the patient can repeat after one hearing. Some persons who use numbers regularly may correctly repeat seven or eight forward. Everyone should be able to repeat at least five. To repeat the numbers in reverse order is more difficult and involves an intellectual process. Most patients can do this one digit less than repeated forward.

Some understanding of the patient's memory may be gained by having the patient repeat an actual current event or a well-known fictional story. Stories may be fabricated to match the background of any patient, thus increasing the likelihood that they will be remembered if there is no problem.

In Korsakow's psychosis there is a gross deficit of memory for recent events of up to half-an-hour beforehand. In addition, there is loss of orientation to space, time, and insight. The patient characteristically fills the memory gap by confabulating (creating imaginary accounts of activities). Such patients cannot recall the recent past, nor can they relate it to the current experience. There is a failure to appreciate the passing of time. When this syndrome is suspected, the examiner can easily lead the patient into confabulation by suggesting that he saw the patient yesterday in a store. The patient may then assure the examiner that he indeed recalls seeing him there, relates how the doctor was dressed, and may go on to relate the details of his purchase.

There is often some decrease in memory associated with aging. This decrease is noted earlier and progresses at a faster rate in patients with Alzheimer's Disease (presenile and senile dementia). Memory is rarely affected by cerebrovascular disease. Alzheimer's Disease is the most common cause of gradual memory loss beyond the age of 50.[3]

6. **Affective state and mood.** Emotion is an affective state of consciousness in which such feelings as joy, sorrow, fear, hate, and love are experienced. Emotions are basic for survival of the individual and the human race. Each external stimulus coming into the brain and every idea arising in it has a cognitive aspect and an affective one. Man uses his large and highly developed cerebrum to inhibit or override the affective aspect much of the time. He can do this for a while, some longer than others; but this cannot be tolerated indefinitely. Man's feeling needs

must be satisfied and his fears must be relieved. Ultimately, these basic drives that go back perhaps millions of years must be addressed. Healthy man achieves a working balance between the two elements of the cerebrum: the cognitive and the affective.

The affective state is the examiner's observation of the patient's apparent feelings during the evaluation. In contrast, the mood reflects the patient's reported subjective feelings.

Facial expression tells the examiner a great deal: whether sadness or elation, anger, anxiety, or absence of feeling. The examiner determines (from observation) if the patient's affect is appropriate for the situation, if there is inordinate variability in moment-to-moment feelings or if the patient is ambivalent (e.g., pathological, simultaneous presence of contradictory feelings directed towards an object or person, such as love and hate for one's spouse). Does the patient show feelings appropriate to the content of speech? Does the patient appear to be "affectively flat," dramatic, or histrionic?

The term mood refers to a prevailing and relatively enduring emotional state. There are many varieties and shades of moods; all can change quickly. The mood of the patient may reflect homesickness and a normal degree of sadness or happiness. It can also reflect pathologically lowered spirits (depression) or pathological elation (mania). When periodic excessive variations occur, the patient is considered cyclothymic. Apathy is a lack of feeling tone. When the mood is one of uneasiness, an uncomfortable, painful, foreboding, subjective feeling, and the cause is known, it would be defined as fear. If the cause of the uneasiness is unknown, it is defined as anxiety. Anxiety can also be produced by toxins, chemicals, and drugs such as adrenalin, ephedrine, amphetamine, nicotine, caffeine and thyroxine, all of which stimulate the sympathetic nervous system. It can also be caused by head injury and/or cerebral disease which diminish the higher centers' control of emotional reactions. Fear can be prominent in delirious states, probably in reaction to hallucinations. In those of the involutional age group fear is sometimes seen in depression.

Emotional instability is a common symptom of diffuse central nervous system lesions. A very slight stimulus may move the patient to laughter or tears (more often the latter) or cause irritation, anger, or apprehension. This is encountered after head injury, massive strokes, in early stages of dementia, and advanced stages of multiple sclerosis. This emotional lability is probably due to impaired control of higher centers over the thalamus and hypothalamus. Emotional instability, when extreme, presents in impulsive actions rather than feelings. This is most often seen in children or adolescents in whom higher control of feelings and actions is incomplete.

Emotional apathy is a general loss of emotional responsiveness without a proportionate intellectual deterioration. This is often seen in post-encephalitic Parkinsonism. A similar state is seen in advanced dementia; patients lose former interests and feelings, and ultimately exist in a vegetative state.

Euphoria is an emotion or a mood characterized by feelings of great cheerfulness and happiness. Alcohol causes this transiently in some people. It often occurs in patients having multiple sclerosis and some other central nervous system diseases; it is poorly understood.

Excitement refers to mental overactivity in which there are intellectual, emotional, and/or psychomotor components. In acute mania all three are simultaneously present as flight of ideas, elation, and psychomotor restlessness. Disordered ideas linked with excitement may be seen in delirious and confusional states, and in catatonic schizophrenia.

Delirium is confusion combined with overexcitement. It can result from head injury, diffuse diseases of the brain, various metabolic diseases, toxins, and drug withdrawal.

Psychomotor restlessness associated with anxiety is seen in agitated depression. An advanced degree of this excited mood is rage; it is seen in aggressive psychopaths.

7. **Intellectual functioning.** Intellectual functioning, or cognition, refers to those psychic processes by which any kind of knowledge is obtained. It includes all aspects of perceiving, remembering, and thinking.

Good intellectual functioning is required for successful adaptation to life. This includes the ability to reason, to express oneself coherently and accurately, and to interpret reality accurately.[4] The ability to relate the details of one's problems is in itself an important test of intellectual functioning.

Many specific abilities can be tested; however all require interpretation considering the patient's social background, education, present situation, and nature of problem. Initial testing and documentation in this area can be regarded as a control against which to measure future improvement or deterioration. Before the physician attempts to examine intellectual functioning, a determination must be made of the patient's ability to listen and to understand a question.

The number of digits forward which the patient can repeat after the examiner gives them at one-per-second is a time-honored test, as is the number of digits backwards which can be repeated. The time required to subtract successive sevens from one hundred (or any given starting number), and the number of errors is also a good base-line against which to judge future function. These tests also measure intelligence and memory as well as attention span and concentration.

The fund of information relating to the patient's social background and formal education requires interpretation (e.g., name five rivers, five cities, the last five presidents). The vocabulary and grammar used should be in keeping with the patient's educational background and status.

A proverb interpretation test is less important and dependable than believed in the past. The same is true regarding the ability to state similarities between items, such as an apple and a banana (answer: both are fruit).[5]

8. **Thought processes.** The normal person has control over a logical and orderly thought process. There may be unexplainable blocking when in the middle of a sentence. Alternatively, ideas may come so fast that there is rapid skipping from one to another in a disjointed or bizarre way. This flight of ideas may be stimulated from internal thought or from the environment. New words may be coined (neologisms), thoughts may have special meanings only to the patient (autistic thinking), ideas may be expressed over and over (perseveration), contiguous thoughts and statements may bear no relationship to each other (loose associations), and the patient may replace memory loss by fantasy or a fabricated reality (confabulation).

9. **Thought content.** It is the content of one's thoughts as expressed in words or nonverbal language that permit the examiner to know the inner life of the patient. The patient may think unceasingly about an unwanted thought (obsession), spend much of his time trying to make a decision, or be preoccupied with a bodily function. The patient may have feelings of worthlessness or of being unworthy to live. The patient may be immobilized by irrational and unrealistic fears or feelings of helplessness and/or hopelessness. The patient's comments may reveal beliefs that are out of keeping with the patient's level of knowledge. Comments may reveal that he is lonely though in the company of friends, or that he is being treated unfairly in the absence of any supportive evidence. The patient may have feelings of being in another world, estranged from self, body, or surroundings. The patient may reveal an intent to harm another person (homicidal) or inflict self-harm (suicidal). Such thoughts always demand careful attention.

The Weschler Adult Intelligence Scale (WAIS) is the standard test for cognitive ability, thought-process, and thought-content. The physician needs a less detailed test requiring less administrative time. The test should be quick, easy to use, and acceptable to patients and testers. Such a test needs to meet the following criteria:

1. Detection and documentation of a cognitive problem alone or in association with other mental problems.
2. Detection of improvement as recovery occurs.
3. Documentation of further deterioration as the disease progresses.
4. Demonstrated reliability and validity.

The Mini-Mental State (MMS) examination consists of eleven questions and requires only five to ten minutes. Its validity and reliability have been documented.[6] It meets the above criteria quite well and is useful in measuring the patient's cognitive ability.

10.   **Disorders of Perception.** Perception refers to a complex process by which one is meaningfully aware of objects, their identity and characteristics, as well as their relationship to other objects and to the patient. Here the definitions of several words are important. To perceive is to become aware of or to gain knowledge of something through one of the senses. An illusion is a misinterpretation of a real sensory experience. A hallucination is a false sensory perception in the absence of actual external stimulus. A hypnagogic experience is a disordered perception occurring in the semiconscious state immediately preceding sleep. A hypnopompic experience is similar except it occurs immediately on awakening. Déjà vu is a sensation of familiarity; that which a first time experience feels as if it has been experienced before. Jamais vu is the opposite, a sensation of strangeness that has been experienced many times, yet feels like a new experience. When disorders of perception are suspected, carefully worded questions are necessary to determine if the patient has had any of these experiences.

Everyone's conception and perception of reality is influenced by past and present experiences, wishes, fears, aspirations, and feelings. Questions for the physician to ask include: is the patient's thinking vulnerable to delusional concepts of the world or self; is the patient suspicious of others; is there a feeling of persecution, surveillance, or control by outside influences only perceived by the patient; is the patient grandiose or demeaning; what is the patient's concept of the future?

11.   **Judgment.** Judgment is a very complex cerebral function. Questions relating to social norms, utilization of funds, and job expectations may reveal that the patient's judgment is bizarre or unrealistic. The patient can be asked what will happen if the electric bill is not paid for six months, or what effect will resigning from a job have on the family. A classic question pertains to finding a sealed letter with an uncancelled stamp on it and asking what the patient would do with it.

12.   **Conversion syndrome.** Psychological stresses in one's life may be translated into disturbances of the special senses and/or the voluntary nervous system. Hysterical blindness and paralysis are examples.

13.   **Somatization.** Emotional disorders may cause somatic complaints (and produce affective equivalents) through physiological changes brought about through the autonomic nervous system (or neuroendocrine system). Irritable colon, diarrhea, muscle contraction, headache, emesis, impotence, frigidity, changes in sexual interest, and disturbed

sleep patterns are examples. The examiner should be alert for the autonomic concomitants of anxiety, dilated pupils, tachycardia, pallor, sweaty palms, and tremor.

14. **Insight.** From the history and on direct questioning the examiner can determine if the patient realizes that there is an emotional or mental problem, and if the need for help is recognized.

Each family physician should evaluate the mental status of a new patient with the same discipline and thoroughness as in examining any organ or body function. Just as one does not do an exhaustive cardiopulmonary evaluation if the patient's complaint is diarrhea, similarly a limited mental status evaluation is sufficient if there is no indication of a mental or emotional problem. Inquiry into the following list of items is suggested as a minimal screening mental status examination:

1. Orientation to person, place, and time
2. Behavior during examination
3. Memory
4. Intellectual functioning
5. Mood
6. Insight

Thus, a brief dictation might be: the patient is oriented to time, place, and person. He is cooperative and gives a good history which reflects a good memory. His intellectual functioning is normal for his background and education. He is emotionally stable and his mood is appropriate. He has good insight into his problem.

A mental status examination requires clinical sensitivity; everyone appreciates tact. To begin by asking a high school principal to count from ten backwards to one could upset a well person. Expressing an interest in the rhythm of his speech (and you should be) makes the question acceptable. Similarly, most questions can be introduced in a manner that will enlist the patient's interest and cooperation.

While the examiner listens to the patient's verbal answers (lyrics), he also watches facial expressions and body movement (melody). The melody is almost always the more reliable communicator of the patient's true feelings. Unverbalized tension states are sometimes communicated through posture, voice tone, pressure of speech, and body movements. When the patient smiles with his mouth but not his eyes, and says he is happy but increases the wringing movements of his hands, the seasoned clinician will explore the problem further. This is where artistry in clinical medicine pays high dividends.

SOME CLINICAL APPLICATIONS

Organic Brain Syndromes

Organic brain syndromes (OBS) refer to direct or indirect effects of diffuse organic disease or dysfunction of the brain resulting in impairment of higher cerebral functions.[7] The term OBS is a convenient clinical term describing a group of behaviors and deficiencies. It is vital that the clinician define the underlying problem or disease which is causing the OBS. Ultimately, effective therapy must be aimed at the etiology of the problem.

Organic brain syndromes are divided into the acute and chronic varieties.[8] In the acute form (AOBS), a confused state develops quickly, even to the development of a frank psychosis. The prime abnormality is an altered state of consciousness. The brain is globally affected with some fluctuation in severity from hour to hour, day to day. The patient is less than normally alert, and has difficulty in focusing attention to answer questions, or to cooperate in the examination. The patient is partially, if not totally, disoriented; and remembers few, if any, of the experiences associated with this state.

The patient's behavior is usually markedly abnormal because of impaired consciousness, difficulty in sorting out sensory inputs, and an abnormal perception of events. Shadows on the wall may be perceived as enemies; strange noises may be very threatening. Ideally, these patients should be in well-lighted and familiar rooms, cared for by people they know. The next best person is a trained attendant who will speak clearly, use simple phrases, and comfort with supportive behavior. It is usual for patients to be more symptomatic after transfer from home to a hospital. Symptoms and behavior fluctuate widely in a 24-hour period, varying with such factors as light, noise, number, and kinds of visitors.

Emotional reactions in AOBS are abnormal and unpredictable. When associated with alcohol or drug abuse, this state is often called delirium or toxic psychosis. Cognition is greatly impaired as evidenced by disorientation, poor memory, poor judgment, difficulty in concentrating or directing one's attention, faulty perception of stimuli, faulty comprehension of words, and faulty reasoning. The patient may be quiet and withdrawn, or acutely disturbed, anxious, excited, and agitated. Paranoid ideas may be expressed in voluble, incoherent speech. The patient may be frightened by visual or auditory hallucinations. Seizures may occur if the AOBS is due to alcohol or drug withdrawal.

Chronic organic brain syndrome (COBS) has the clinical appearance of dementia associated with depressed consciousness. Its onset and development are very insidious and slowly but steadily progressive. Errors of orientation and memory are more noteworthy than in AOBS.

In chronic OBS the first change to be observed may be in the personality of the patient. Affect may become blunted and shallow as the patient responds less to pleasant and disagreeable comments, events, or situations than in the past. To the embarrassment of family and friends, the patient may become less discreet in language and behavior. Some of the behavior may be impulsive by nature, manifesting itself in angry outbursts, vulgarity, and indiscreet sexual behavior. The patient may change from a pattern of neatness and punctuality to one of personal untidiness and tardiness, and show a lack of concern about such behavior.

The patient with chronic organic brain syndrome (COBS) has impaired memory (recent more than remote), faulty orientation to time and place, difficulty in concentrating and directing his attention. He has difficulty solving arithmetic problems, even in comprehending the problem. The patient's speech may be rambling, incoherent, and repetitious.

Many patients with chronic OBS have no insight into the above changes. They probably utilize the psychological defense mechanism of denial and some will confabulate to fill in the gaps in their memories. Other patients who retain some insight into their problem are not as fortunate. They feel great distress and embarrassment when they cannot answer questions or perform tasks that would have been easily accomplished at an earlier time.

Some patients suffer from depression as their abilities decline. A few will develop paranoid ideas as their declining intellectual abilities curtail their daily living activities.

Depression

Depression is one of the most common problems encountered by the family physician. In evaluating mental status, it is important to separate ordinary sadness from depression. Every person experiences "the blues," loneliness, and worries. This is usually short-lived and can be called "reactive sadness." The person experiencing reactive sadness can continue to function and feels better when reassured. On the other hand, the depressed person cannot function normally, depression lasts longer (at least one month), and even if circumstances change for the better, the depression does not go away. The following diagnostic triad for depression is useful:

1. There is a pervasive disturbance of mood characterized by sadness, crying, discouragement, anxiety, and irritability.
2. There is a change in the patient's self-perception, his environment, and his future. The patient sees and feels himself as helpless, hopeless, worthless, and guilty (for which there is no relief or forgiveness). He experiences lowered self-esteem, loss of interest in usual activities and happenings in the home, and a view that the future is worse than the present. There may be suicidal thoughts and plans.
3. Depression affects the functioning of the body (vegetative signs) as well as the mood and thoughts of the mind. The most common vegetative change is a sleep disturbance characterized by early morning awakening. Depressed feelings are worse early in the day and lessen as the day goes on (diurnal variation). Appetite loss and usually a corresponding weight decrease occur; constipation is often associated. The patient complains of tachycardia and fatigue. There is decreased interest in sex and ability to function satisfactorily in this area.

When depression is suspected, in addition to the above triad, the following clues should be sought in the mental status evaluation:

4. The depression may have been initiated by a significant loss. This may be a spouse, a dear friend, income, self-esteem, or status in the community.
5. There may be a history of previous depressed episodes. The history will less often reveal one or more episodes of mania.
6. There is a higher incidence of depression, mania, alcoholism, and antisocial behavior in the family members.

It is not enough to determine that the patient is depressed; the underlying reason should be sought. Depression can be caused by infections (especially influenza), organic diseases of the brain, and malignancies. It can occur as a reaction to a loss, such as self-respect or a loved one. It can be a neurotic reaction to internal difficulties and to feelings of guilt or anger. Depression is the predominant feature of involutional melancholia and is often associated with agitation.

The sensitive and intuitive physician can support the depressed patient by moving a chair closer to symbolize sharing of the problem. The physician may reach out and touch the patient to strengthen this gesture. The physician will sense and should respect the effort required for the depressed patient to mobilize sufficient psychomotor energy to get out of bed, to dress, to discuss troubles, and reveal feelings. Let the patient know you understand the strain this represents, and express appreciation for this effort to encourage cooperation as mental status evaluation proceeds.

Stoical people who become depressed have a special problem; they believe it is unacceptable to cry. The physician's encouragement for patients to behave as they feel, and the recognition that it takes courage to open up to feelings, can constitute "permission" for the patient to cry and ventilate pent-up feelings. The patient may then be able and willing to provide more information for the mental status evaluation.

A useful self-rating depression scale (SDS) consisting of 20 questions was first published by Zung in 1965.[9] The individual items indicate the area affected (affect, physical, psychomotor disturbance, psychological) while aggregate scores express the degree of depression. This is a good test to use when the mental status evaluation uncovers depression. This is discussed more fully in Chapter 13.

Hysteria

The family physician caring for the patient over an extended period knows the family as well as the community and is in an ideal position to recognize hysterical patients and promptly diagnose the complaint. This can avoid the performance of many hospital tests which medicalize the complaint and support neurotic response to life-stress.

Under stress it seems that certain psycho-physiological elements become separated (mental dissociation) from the conscious life of the patient. Whatever is responsible for this entity is inborn or develops at an early age. It is seen far more frequently in women than men and most often becomes clinically manifest in second or third decades. Family physicians should be very cautious in making this diagnosis to explain new symptoms seen in persons past forty. Patients having been erroneously labeled hysterical are not infrequently later shown to have multiple sclerosis, temporal lobe disease, depression, or dementia.

The challenge for the clinician is to determine the meaning and purpose of the symptom to the patient. A patient may be confronted with a conflict between two opposing wishes. The patient may be in a situation in which a desired course of action conflicts with a sense of duty or self-respect. Development of the hysterical symptom unconsciously solves the conflict, though at the price of developing a neurotic disability. For example, a college student with an excellent past academic record feels threatened by a coming examination for which she has poorly prepared. Paralysis of the right arm is developed and the examination cannot be taken. Self-respect is maintained, the record is not spoiled, and blame is not assessed. A more complex example follows. A girl was compelled to abandon her work to care for her invalid mother. Hysterical paralysis of her right hand prevented her from doing housework; assistance had to be obtained to look after herself and her mother. Her hysterical illness saved her from unpleasant duty and preserved her self-respect; she felt that no one could blame her for being ill. At the same time she ceased to do any work at all, unconsciously revenging herself on her exacting parent, and creating an object of sympathy to those with whom she came in contact. This example shows how the hysterical symptom may serve multiple purposes.

The diagnosis of hysteria requires three criteria:

1. The presence of signs of hysteria, i.e., the symptoms and findings do not correspond to the anatomy and physiology of the body.
2. There is an absence of signs of disease which might explain the symptoms and findings.
3. A usual motive for the hysterical episode can be uncovered during the mental status examination.

Since hysterical symptoms develop as the result of stress or a problem, they will usually subside as the stress resolves itself, recurring when stress returns or another stress situation develops. Thus, the hysterical symptom tends to be transient and intermittent, suggesting repeated bouts of illness.

REFERENCES

1. Lurie HJ: *Clinical Psychiatry for the Primary Care Physician.* Roche Laboratories, 1976
2. Weitzel WD, Morgan DW, Guyden TE, Robinson JA: Toward a more efficient mental status exam. Arch Gen Psychiatry 28:215–218, 1973
3. Lord TLL, Walton JN: *Diseases of the Nervous System.* 7th ed. London: Oxford University Press, 1969, pp. 989–993
4. Adams RD, Victor M: *Principles of Neurology.* 1st ed. New York: McGraw-Hill Book Company, 1977, pp. 5–6
5. Andreasen NC: Reliability and validity of proverb interpretation to assess mental status. Comp Psychiatry 18:465–472, 1977
6. Folstein MF, Folstein SE, McHugh PR: Mini-mental state: A practical method for grading the cognitive state of patients for the clinician. J Psychiat Res 12:189–198, 1975
7. Duboxsky SL, Weissberg MP: *Clinical Psychiatry in Primary Care.* Baltimore: Williams & Wilkins Company, 1978
8. Harvey AM, Johns RJ, Owens AH, Jr, Ross RS: *The Principles and Practice of Medicine.* 19th ed. New York: Appleton-Century-Crofts, 1976, pp. 1, 641–642
9. Zung WW: Self-rating depression scale. Arch of General Psychology 12:63, 1965

CHAPTER 12

SELF-MONITORING BY PATIENTS

JOHN L. SHELTON AND GERALD M. ROSEN

Physicians often ask patients about behavior. For example, diabetic and obese patients are frequently asked to recall daily diet patterns. Tension headache sufferers estimate the frequency, duration, and intensity of pain; other patients may report their exercise patterns, the number of cigarettes smoked, or their daily consumption of alcohol. In other instances, parents are asked to describe their children's eating and sleeping patterns, the number of nights of bedwetting, or the number of temper tantrums in a day. In these and numerous other situations, the physician relies upon a patient's recall of behavioral events.

A patient's recall of behavioral events can provide useful data for the physician. Yet, reliance upon patient recall has its limitations. As time passes between a behavioral event and its reporting, the accuracy of recall is likely to diminish. Recall and global estimates of a behavioral event are also subject to distortion and bias; usually in the direction of a desirable response. As a result, the physician cannot be certain if the obese patient accurately recalls caloric intake, if the married patient accurately reports sexual satisfaction, or if a parent describes developmental history.

Recall of a behavioral event is also limited insofar as the patient is unaware of the event or critical factors which affect it. Simply stated, most patients do not take the time to pay close attention to everyday changes in their behavior. Patients also fail to observe relationships between their behavior and environmental factors that influence them. The family physician is familiar with these situations. An obese patient is unable to recall pertinent information in response to the question, "What situations or emotional events seem to increase your desire to eat?" Headache patients report having headaches all day, but cannot pinpoint those times of day when pain is greatest. And frequently parents are unaware of the immediate consequences of their child's temper tantrums.

Because of limitations inherent in patient recall, physicians have employed more systematic methods for obtaining accurate information about behavioral events. The purpose of this chapter is to illustrate such methods by discussing approaches to patient self-monitoring.

PATIENT'S SELF-MONITORING OF BEHAVIOR

Self-monitoring refers to systematic or controlled behavioral observations planned with a professional and conducted by the patient in his or her own environment. When properly performed, self-monitoring allows the physician to observe patient behavior throughout the day, and can serve as useful assessment functions during both diagnosis and treatment. Initially, it can help to define a patient's complaint and provide data on the frequency, duration, and intensity of a problem. In the diagnostic phase of data collection, self-monitoring can clarify the relationship between the patient's environment and disability or illness. A systematic observation of eating, cigarette smoking, temper tantrums, or other behavior takes place; it becomes possible to identify relationships between that behavior and the environment, and to plan treatment strategies. For millions of Americans, a football game on television is a powerful cue that initiates overeating. For these people, television viewing has been so frequently paired with eating that the two have become temporally linked. The result is that television watching becomes almost impossible without a sandwich in hand. Self-monitoring allows the identification of such controlling cues which can yield control of the behavior they activate. Controlling the amount of television watching can actually influence the amount of food consumed.

In a similar manner, self-monitoring can clarify the consequences of a behavior which may be serving to maintain the problem of interest. Familiar examples of such relationships are the child who gets candy after a temper tantrum, the dissatisfied spouse who avoids sex by having a headache, and the low-back-pain patient who no longer goes to work.

These and countless other sickness-related behaviors are encouraged and supported by the favorable consequences immediately following their occurrence.

Consideration of self-monitoring can clarify both the environmental antecedents that elicit behavior and the consequences that maintain it; it is useful to think of the "A-B-C" model of behavior. Within this model, behavior "B" is viewed as being a function of eliciting antecedent stimuli "A," and the consequences following "C." A clarification of the various relationships between A, B, and C is known as a functional analysis of behavior. In many cases, a full understanding of a patient problem and appropriate planning of a treatment strategy require that such an analysis be conducted. An example will illustrate this point.

Case Illustration

Robert consulted his physician about his weight problem which had gradually gotten worse over the years. Robert's weight, 284 pounds, was now a threat to his health and his occupation. Through an interview, Dr. King determined that Robert had experienced a long history of abortive attempts to lose weight. Virtually every crash diet imaginable had been tried, found wanting, and then discarded. Robert and his doctor agreed that his weight should be 175 pounds.

Robert's physician attempted to treat the problem by focusing on the environmental cues that stimulated overeating, plus the eating behavior itself. To accomplish these ends, he asked Robert to keep careful track of his "B," the eating behavior, and the situations in which it occurred ("A"). To assist in this task, Dr. King provided Robert with a thumb-operated mechanical counter recording behavior up to 999 units. Robert was instructed to click the counter every time he took a mouthful. He was also provided with a standardized recording sheet similar to that illustrated in Figure 12-1.

The resultant data allowed Dr. King and his patient to determine under what circumstances eating occurred and the consequences that followed. The assessment revealed the following facts. Robert was consuming an average of 340 mouthfuls a day, as compared to about 150 for the typical 175-pound man. Obviously Robert's "B" was out of control. The situations in which Robert ate were typically meal-centered, (i.e., Robert did not snack). An analysis of what Robert ate also revealed a fairly normal pattern of eating behavior. Robert did not consume excess sugars or carbohydrates; he simply ate too much. Most relevant to the planning of a treatment program was finding that consequences of eating were maintaining the problem. Robert's records revealed that his wife (Grace) had developed a long-standing habit of cooking more than was required. Further, if Robert did not overeat, she became hurt and angry, feeling that her cooking had not been satisfactory.

In effect, the behavioral analysis revealed that Grace, not Robert, needed treatment. By asking what are the consequences which encourage

Name _____

DAY _____	(B) Type and Amount	Eating Habits (A) Place, Persons, Activity	(C) Consequences
Morning 8:00 9:00 10:00 11:00 12:00			
Afternoon 1:00 2:00 3:00 4:00 5:00 6:00			
Evening 7:00 8:00 9:00 10:00 11:00 & Later			

FIGURE 12-1.   A diet monitoring form.

overeating and/or discourage moderation, it was possible to identify controlling factors and then arrange for a meeting with Robert and his wife. Functional analysis of behavior and identification of the A-B-C sequence led Dr. King to formulate a treatment intervention differing greatly from binge eating or overeating while watching television. The major focus of Robert's treatment involved retraining Grace to cook differently and respond to Robert in new ways.

Once treatment has begun, self-monitoring performs another vital function. Aside from aiding in the diagnostic phase of treatment, self-monitoring can provide important data regarding the impact of the treatment intervention. In this second function, incoming data regarding the effectiveness of treatment provide the basis for making changes in original treatment plans.

SELF-MONITORING SYSTEMS

There are numerous methods or formats that can be used to accomplish accurate and informative self-recording. The method used by a physician will depend on the needs of a particular patient, and questions of immediate concern. While the majority of self-monitoring formats can be designed in the office, standardized formats are available and may be desirable when large numbers of patients suffer from the same basic problem. Recent publications list scores of commercially available formats.[1-2]

Various formats that can be tailored to particular patient problems will be briefly presented here. These examples are illustrative of general strategies. In practice, the formats will be varied and combined to answer whatever questions are relevant at a particular time.

Frequency Counts

A simple frequency count is often sufficient to learn more about a behavior of interest. How many headaches occur in the day? How many unreasonable requests are made by a child? How many nights a week does the patient take sleep medication? All that is required to develop a self-monitoring system answering these questions is a definition of target behavior and the time period of interest. While a small piece of paper is

NAME _____		WEEK OF _____					
Activity	**Mon**	**Tues**	**Wed**	**Thur**	**Fri**	**Sat**	**Sun**
Went Walking							
Visited Friends							
Shopped							
Went Sight-Seeing							
Rode Bus							

FIGURE 12-2.   Frequency recording for treatment of chronic pain.

PATIENT _____   DATE _____

Please shade in the areas of your body where you
are currently experiencing pain.

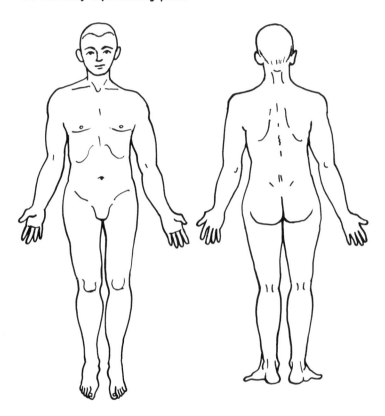

FIGURE 12-3.   Rating scale for number of painful areas on the body.
(Adapted from Fordyce et al.: Behavioral Methods for Chronic Pain and
Illness. St. Louis: The C. V. Mosby Company, 1976.)

the simplest way to record frequency counts, more novel methods have
been devised. In one report, a patient moved a toothpick from one com-
partment of her purse to another each time targeted behavior occurred.[3]
Another person transferred pennies from one pocket to another representing each occurrence of the targeted problem. A variety of counting
devices can also be used. Golf-counters are readily available, as are the
price-tallying counters sold in supermarkets.

   Two examples of self-monitoring systems used with chronic pain
patients are provided in Figures 12-2 and 12-3.[4] In the first example, a

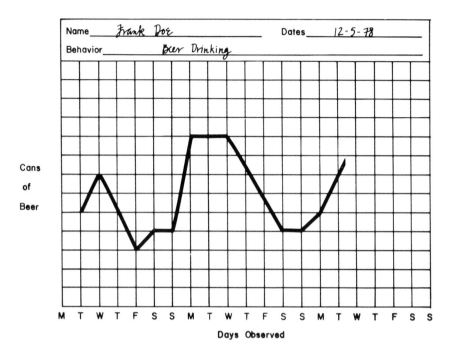

Name ___Frank Doe_____ Dates ___12-5-78___

Behavior _____Beer Drinking_____

Cans
of
Beer

M T W T F S S M T W T F S S M T W T F S S

Days Observed

FIGURE 12-4. Using graph paper to record the frequency of cans of beer consumed.

patient records the number or frequency of various activities that may need to be increased in later treatment. In the second example, the number of areas in the body where pain is experienced can be shaded by the patient on provided drawings. The physician can then count the number of areas shaded; as treatment progresses, the number of shaded areas should diminish.

Some physicians find keeping graph paper in the office convenient to assist patients in self-monitoring. The top of each sheet has space for the physician to write particular behavioral events of interest. In Figure 12-4 the patient has monitored beer-drinking frequency. This graph shows that Mr. Doe drinks nearly every day, averaging six cans of beer. It would be just as easy for the patient to track cigarettes, problems with a spouse, and children's temper tantrums.

Although a frequency format is direct and simple to administer, in particular cases one may want to obtain additional information. In such cases it can be useful to have an open-ended space included for general comments. Figure 12-5 uses data displayed in Figure 12-4 and presents an alternative format with additional comments.

Figure 12-6 shows an all-purpose frequency format which can be

Behavior	Beer Drinking	Name Mr. Black
Date	**Frequency**	**Comments**
1	╫╫╫ ╫╫╫	Stopped off at bar with working buddies
2	11	Very slow day, worked in yard
3	╫╫╫ ╫╫╫ 1	Attended Seahawk game (we lost)
4	╫╫╫ 1111	Watched Monday night football—drank a lot
5	111	Had my beer with dinner
6	1	Had beer for dinner
7	╫╫╫	Went bowling
8	╫╫╫ ╫╫╫	Stopped at bar with gang

FIGURE 12-5. An open-ended frequency recording system. Occasionally one may want to obtain more data than just the frequency of an event. This format illustrates how this may be done.

adapted to any behavior occurring five times or less daily. Frequency count formats can be expanded to monitor additional aspects of a targeted behavior so that a behavioral functional analysis is possible. Figure 12-1 provides a dieting form that helps to clarify the antecedents and consequences controlling eating behaviors. The form asks the patient to monitor frequency of eating, the time of day it occurs, the types and quantity of food ingested, the people or situations that may be eliciting eating behaviors, and the consequences resulting from eating. A similar format can be used to study other problem behaviors. For example, when applied to child behavior problems, a parent could record the nature and extent of a temper tantrum in the first column. Instead of discussing place, person, or cues eliciting eating, the parent would record what activity the child was engaged in at the time of the tantrum. Instead of noting if satisfied feelings of fullness or guilt over eating ensued, the parent would note how the temper tantrum was dealt with, such as punishment or buying a toy.

Name _____   Behavior ____ Relaxation _____

Week _____

	Saturday				
Friday					
Thursday					
Wednesday					
Tuesday					
Monday					
Sunday					

FIGURE 12-6.   A frequency recording for more than six behaviors a day.

Duration Measures

While frequency counts are useful to record discrete target behaviors, the duration of a particular behavioral event may be an important variable. Duration may be self-monitored by means of a stopwatch; several commercially available wrist-watches now have a stopwatch accessory. Electric clocks that are specially wired or chess clocks can also be used to monitor the duration of activities like television watching or study time.[5] When the target behavior is occurring, the switch remains in the on position, permitting the self-recording clock to accumulate the duration measures. An example of a duration recording of pain behavior is provided in Figure 12-7.

Combination Recording Systems

By combining the two basic systems previously described, one can design an almost unlimited number of self-monitoring formats tailor-made to a patient. For example, with little additional planning, the basic idea of duration monitoring can be altered or combined with other recording methods to measure several dimensions of a given problem. One example of such a format, useful for the treatment of chronic pain, has been developed by Fordyce and his associates.[6] The Activity Diary is illustrated in Figure 12-8. In order to use this self-monitoring format successfully, the patient is asked to record data several times during the day. After completing each daily diary the patient then totals the hours of the three activity categories. The total hours spent sitting, walking, and reclining should add up to 24 each day.

Figure 12-9 illustrates a similar format designed for the treatment of headaches. This assessment card provides a simple self-monitoring system for tracking the duration and intensity of headaches, as well as the medication taken to manage the pain. Totaling the number of cards completed on a given day provides a frequency count.

Additional self-monitoring formats for tension-related problems are illustrated in Figures 12-10 and 12-11 and are taken from a relaxation training program.[7] The first form was developed so as to be adaptable to most any tension-related problem. Figure 12-10 shows this form as it was completed by a patient with tension headaches and family-related issues. The ratings were made on a ten-point tension scale, where zero equals totally relaxed and ten equals maximum patient tension. Whatever scale a physician chooses to use with the patient, the end points of that scale should be clearly defined. It can be observed that situational analyses are possible in this type of form. For example, as the patient recorded her

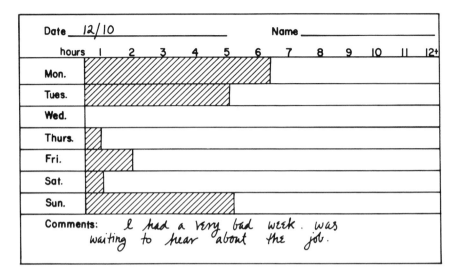

FIGURE 12-7.   A duration recording of tension headaches.

tension regarding picking her son up at school, it became evident that the extent of traffic was an important factor. The "kids getting in her hair" was a determining factor surrounding tension over dinner.

Figure 12-11 illustrates a form that can be used when general feelings of tension exist, rather than a specifically focused physical complaint or problem situation. The patient rates peak tension level on the same ten-point scale as above. Two-hour time intervals are defined and whenever a high rating is made, the patient comments on possible contributing factors. This form can be extremely useful with patients complaining of nonspecific general tension problems. The form also illustrates how daily averages, as well as averages for each time interval, can be computed. In this way it may be possible to identify with the patient particular days, time periods, or situations contributing to high tension points.

ENHANCING THE ACCURACY OF SELF-MONITORING

The accuracy of self-monitored data can vary dramatically depending on the situation, the behavior being monitored, and the recording methods used.[8] The physician asking patients to self-monitor a behavioral event should consider the following guidelines.

1.   Prepare the patient for self-monitoring. The likelihood of obtaining reliable self-monitored data begins in the office with thorough patient

DAY _Tuesday_   DATE _6/15/76_

	Sitting		Walking & Standing		Reclining		Medications		Pain Level
	Major Activity	Time	Major Activity	Time	Activity	Time	Amount	Type	(0-10)
12-1am					Sleep	60			
1-2					Sleep	60			
2-3					Sleep	60			
3-4					Sleep	60			
4-5					Sleep	60			
5-6					Sleep	60			
6-7					Sleep	60			
7-8	Eating	15	Cooking	15	Sleep	30	10 M.	Darvon	6
8-9	Reading	60							3
9-10	T.V.	60					2 TAB	Tylenol (325 mg.)	1
10-11	T.V.	60							0
11-12					Rest T.V.	60			0
12-1pm	Eating	30	Cooking	30					2
1-2	T.V.	45	Laundry	15					3
2-3	Reading	60					2 TAB	Tylenol (325 mg.)	3
3-4	Visiting	45	Ironing	15					1
4-5	T.V.	30			Rest	30	10 mg	Darvon	4
5-6	Eating	30	Cooking	30					1
6-7	T.V.	45	Dishes	15					0
7-8	Telephone	15	Cleaning	15	Rest T.V.	30			6
8-9					Rest T.V.	60	5 mg	Valium	6
9-10					Reading	60			0
10-11					Sleep	60			
11-12					Sleep	60			

Total Hours ➡ SITTING= 8¼   WALKING= 2¼   RECLINING= 13¼

Pain Scale :
0 = no pain
10 = unbearable

(Hours Sitting + Hours Walking + Hours Reclining = 24 Hours)

FIGURE 12-8.   Comprehensive duration recording system. (Adapted from Fordyce et al.: Behavioral Methods for Chronic Pain and Illness. St. Louis: The C. V. Mosby Company, 1976.

preparation. This starts with a discussion of the benefits achieved by accurate assessment of a problem. Next, easily observed and counted behaviors should be chosen. Finally, the entire sequence of recording a behavioral event should be role-played or rehearsed with the patient until the patient can discriminate instances of target behavior and record their occurrence.

2. Keep assignment manageable. It is generally wise to begin self-monitoring with relatively simple, high frequency response classes. Behaviors that only occur once a month run the risk of not being counted because the patient has forgotten what to count. Even when multiple problems exist, it is best to limit the self-monitored behavior to three or less. Self-monitoring should not be so time consuming or cumbersome that it results in noncompliance.

3. Select an unobtrusive and convenient recording method. It is important to select a recording instrument or system that is always available where and when the behavioral event of interest is likely to occur. When possible, it is helpful to provide the patient with a standardized record-

---

HEADACHE INCIDENT CARD

Name _____   Date _____

1. Start
   _____AM
   _____PM

2. Intensity Rating (circle one)

   0 = no pain at all
   10 = worst possible pain

   0   1   2   3   4   5   6   7   8   9   10

3. Medication:

   _____

   _____

4. End
   _____AM
   _____PM

FIGURE 12-9.   A self-assessment method for headache.

DAY OF THE WEEK	PROBLEM 1 Headaches		PROBLEM 2 Driving Johnny to School		PROBLEM 3 Preparing Dinner	
	Rating	Comments	Rating	Comments	Rating	Comments
MONDAY Jan. 14	8	Started - 9 a.m. Lasted 1 hr. Took 2 aspirin	6	Johnny got to bed late. Was irritable in morning.	8	Got a late start - trouble with kids after school.
TUESDAY 15	5 / 7	9:30 a.m. 1/2 hr. 1 aspirin 6:08 p.m. 1 hr. 1 aspirin	7	Johnny was O.K. but traffic was bad.	9	Trouble with kids.
WEDNESDAY 16	3	9 p.m. 1/2 hr. no medicine	4	Light traffic.	7	Got home late - kids acting up.
THURSDAY 17			4	Light traffic.	8	Trouble with kids.
FRIDAY 18	9	5:00 p.m. 1 hr. 2 aspirin	8	Heavy traffic.	4	Got home early - kids out of the way.
SATURDAY 19	10 / 7	3:00 p.m. 2 hr. 2 1/2 aspirin 7:30 p.m. 1 hr. 2 aspirin			2	Kids tired from day at park - no problem.
SUNDAY 20					4	Kids restless.
AVERAGES:		Headache 1 per day. They lasted 1 hour and my taking averaged 7.0. Averaged 1.5 aspirin per headache.		Driving to school - every weekday. Average rating was 5.8. Tension is a function of traffic.		Preparing dinner - tension high about every day. Average rating was 5.9. Kids behavior is responsible.

FIGURE 12-10. Assessment form for physical complaints and problem situations. (From Gerald Rosen: The Relaxation Book: An Illustrated Self-Help Program. © 1977, pp. 23, 25. Reprinted by permission of Prentice-Hall, Inc., Englewood Cliffs, N.J.

SELF-MONITORING FOR GENERAL TENSION

TIME/DAY	M	T	W	TH	F	S	SU	COMMENTS	AVERAGES
8:00 to 10:00 a.m.	4	5	3	4	3	1	1		3.8
10:00– noon	1	3	1	7	3	2	1	Thursday (7): called car mechanic.	2.6
noon– 2:00 p.m.	2	3	2	3	4	3	1		2.6
2:00– 4:00 p.m.	4	4	5	4	4	2	1		3.4
4:00– 6:00 p.m.	6	8	4	8	9	2	2	Monday (6): kids home and housecleaning wasn't done. Tuesday (8): long lines at grocery store. Thursday (8) and Friday (9): housecleaning not done.	5.6
6:00– 8:00 p.m.	4	3	3	5	6	3	3	Friday (6): tense about entertaining guests.	3.9
8:00– 10:00 p.m.	2	3	1	3	3	4	2		2.6
10:00– 12:00 p.m.	2	1	–	2	2	3	–		2.2

AVERAGES: 3.1, 4.1, 2.7, 4.5, 4.2, 2.7, 1.7

WRITE IN THIS LEFT-HAND COLUMN, TWO HOUR TIME BLOCKS

FIGURE 12-11. Assessment form for recording general feelings of tension. (From Gerald Rosen: The Relaxation Book: An Illustrated Self-Help Program. © 1977, pp. 23, 25. Reprinted by permission of Prentice-Hall, Inc., Englewood Cliffs, N.J.)

ing format—diary forms such as those illustrated earlier, hand counters, the penny system, the toothpick system, or some other prearranged format. Naturally, the more difficult, inconvenient, or embarrassing a recording format, the less likely patient compliance will be.

4.   Reinforce the patient for accurate records. Several research articles[9, 10, 11] have shown that reinforcing the patient for accurate self-monitoring makes a significant difference in the quality of data obtained. One way to reinforce the patient's efforts is to have the office staff or nurse call the patient shortly after the self-monitoring assignment was made. Subsequent meetings between the patient and physician should begin with a discussion of the recording efforts and patient insights.

5.   Focus on positive events. In order for self-monitoring to be inherently reinforcing to the patient a positive behavioral event should be chosen for observation. Thus, a cigarette smoker could not only record the number of cigarettes smoked (a negative event), but could also track the number of times these urges were resisted (a positive event). Similarly, if a parent and child decide to track the number of the child's temper tantrums, they would benefit by also tracking the number of times the child shows good behavior.

6.   Include accuracy checks by others. Self-monitoring has been shown to be more accurate when self-observers are aware that their accuracy is being monitored by another.[12] This can be accomplished by occasional calls to a spouse or parent. Such an intervention is especially appropriate for children. Not surprisingly, adults are more accurate at self-observation than are children.[13] A physician interested in a child's report of behavior would do well to have a corroborating report from a parent.

It should be noted that when an accuracy check is obtained from someone in addition to the patient, permission must be obtained from the patient.

7.   Recording should be immediate. It is best to have patients record a behavioral event when it occurs, rather than later. In one study, recordings made immediately after a behavior occurred were significantly more accurate than recordings made at the end of the day, or at the end of a week.[14] This is not surprising; daily or weekly estimates depend on recall. Problems associated with memory loss or distortion were previously discussed.

8.   The reactivity of self-monitoring can be explained. It has been demonstrated that the act of self-monitoring can affect the behavior being observed.[15] Fortunately, from a therapeutic point of view, this effect is usually desirable. Desirable behaviors tend to increase during self-monitoring periods and undesirable behaviors tend to decrease. Such changes, in all likelihood, are associated with an increase in the patient's

awareness of his or her behavior and a high motivation to change. To the extent that a physician wishes accurate data uncontaminated by the reactivity effect, it is best to inform patients of this phenomenon. The physician can inform the patient that it is important to have accurate information about current patterns of behavior, so that treatment effects can be properly evaluated. This may help to postpone initial changes in behavior levels.

Because of the direction of the reactivity effect, some physicians may wish to maximize the initial changes that occur as a consequence of self-monitoring. However, studies have found that the therapeutic effects associated with self-observation are weak and short lived.[16] Without a more comprehensive treatment program, the behavior problem usually returns to preassessment levels after several weeks.[17, 18] Thus, self-monitoring is a useful adjunct of treatment, but is no substitute for a program of effective intervention.

CONCLUSIONS

There are numerous occasions where the evaluation of illness and disabilities can be facilitated by a thorough assessment of relevant behaviors. On such occasions, the physician's reliance on the patient's recall of behavioral events may be insufficient. Rather, the physician and patient would come to a more adequate assessment of the particular problem if the patient spent a period of time self-monitoring the events in question. Various formats are available to aid physicians who plan a self-monitoring system for specific patient problems. These formats allow for monitoring various dimensions of behavior including frequency, intensity, and duration. It is also possible to conduct a systematic functional analysis to clarify the eliciting conditions and reinforcing consequences of a particular behavior.

To ensure accurate self-monitoring, it is important that the physician rehearse the details of the recording system with the patient. Clearly defined behaviors, an easy and portable recording system, and a focus on positive behavioral events will help to enhance reliability.

REFERENCES

1. Mash E, Terdal L: *Behavioral Therapy Assessment.* New York: Springer Publishing Company, 1976
2. Ciminero A, Calhoun KS, Adams HE: *Handbook of Behavioral Assessment.* New York: John Wiley and Sons, 1977

3. Mahoney MJ: Self reward and self monitoring techniques for weight control. Beh Ther 5:48–57, 1974

4. Fordyce WE: *Behavioral Methods for Chronic Pain and Illness.* St. Louis: The C. V. Mosby Company, 1976

5. Kazdin AE: "Self-Monitoring and Behavior Change." In: Mahoney MJ, Thoresen SC: *Self-Control: Power to the Person.* Monterey: Brooks-Cole, 1974

6. Fordyce WE, Brena S, DeLateur B, Holcombe S, Loeser J: Diagnostic judgments of chronic pain and MMPI and activity level measures. J Appl Beh Anal, in press

7. Rosen, GM: *The Relaxation Book.* Englewood Cliffs: Prentice-Hall, 1977

8. Thoresen CE, Mahoney MJ: *Behavioral Self Control.* Monterey: Brooks-Cole, 1974

9. Kazdin AE: Reactive self-monitoring: The effects of response desirability, goal setting and feedback. J Consult Clin Psychol 42:704–16, 1974

10. Lipinshi DP, Nelson RO: The reactivity and unreliability of self-recording. J Consult Clin Psychol 42:118, 1974

11. Risely TR, Hart B: Developing correspondence between the non-verbal and verbal behavior. J Appl Beh Anal, 1:267, 1968

12. Mattos RL: A manual counter for recording multiple behavior. J Appl Beh Anal, 1:130, 1968

13. Johnson SJ, While G: Self-observation as an agent of behavioral change. Beh Ther, 2:488–97, 1971

14. Karoly P, Doyle WW: Effects of outcome expectancy and timing of self monitoring on cigarette smoking. J Clin Psychol 31:351–55, 1975

15. Hay LR, Hay WM, Angle HV: The reactivity of self recording: A case report of a drug abuser. Beh Ther, in press

16. Hammen JW, Glass DR: Depression, activity, and evaluation of reinforcement. J Abnorm Psychol 84:718–21, 1975

17. McLaughlin JG, Nay WR: Treatment of trichotillomania using positive coverants and response cost: A case report. Beh Ther 6:87–91, 1975

18. Mahoney MJ: The self management of covert behavior: A case study. Beh Ther 2:575–78, 1971

CHAPTER 13

PSYCHOLOGICAL TESTING

WILLIAM R. PHILLIPS AND GERALD M. ROSEN

Psychological tests sample a set of patient behaviors in a standardized manner. In many ways, these tests are analogous to common clinical laboratory tests. Both rely upon standardized techniques for collecting, evaluating, and recording relevant information. Clinical laboratory and psychological tests can be evaluated on the basis of their reliability and validity. Both approaches permit comparison of an individual's results with appropriate reference groups of healthy and ill individuals. Finally, each test form requires the physician to make sound clinical decisions on the basis of a broader data base. Whether it is a complete blood count, sedimentation rate, or Minnesota Multiphasic Personality Inventory, test results only contribute to clinical judgment and cannot replace it. This chapter considers the types of tests available, introduces the reader to instruments frequently used in medical settings, and discusses directions for the incorporation into clinical practice of these potentially useful tools.

COMMON PSYCHOLOGICAL TESTS

Psychological tests can be categorized in a number of ways. They can be divided into tests designed for group and for individual administration.

TABLE 13-1.   Commonly Used Psychological Tests

Rank	Test	Uses
1	Minnesota Multiphasic Personality Inventory	Objective personality inver..ory for general assessment
2	Denver Developmental Screening Test	Objective inventory of tasks to assess infant and child developmental levels
3	Zung Self-Rating Depression Scale	Short objective format for assessing level of depression
4	Wechsler Adult Intelligence Scale	Objective series of tasks yielding estimate of intelligence for adults
5	Wechsler Intelligence Scale for Children	Objective test for assessing intelligence levels for children
6	Beck Depression Inventory	Short objective format for assessing level of depression
7	Rotter Incomplete Sentence Blank	Projective type test for assessing aspects of a patient's personality and attitudes

There are tests that patients complete on their own and those requiring the skills of a trained psychometrist. Many tests are objective, offering true-false choices or providing questions requiring a single correct answer. Other tests are interpretive or projective, because they provide ambiguous or open-ended stimuli to which patients make idiosyncratic responses.

Categorizing these tests in terms of their intended function is of greatest interest to the family physician. Some tests measure general abilities such as intelligence level, while others measure specific or more limited skills. Tests are available to measure levels of achievement, or to assess basic aptitudes and potential for achievement. Objective personality tests such as the Minnesota Multiphasic Personality Inventory provide global assessments of personality function; as do projective personality tests such as the Rorschach Inkblots, or the Thematic Apperception Test (TAT). Additional psychological tests have been constructed to assess a variety of specific attributes including depression, anxiety, life stresses, marital satisfaction, and vocational interests. Indeed, if a physician has a question about behavior, there is probably a psychological test that can help assess the issue.

The sheer number of psychological tests makes it impossible to attempt a complete survey within a single chapter. The purpose of this chapter will be to focus on tests currently used with some frequency in family practice residency programs. Examples will be presented of psychological tests that already appear useful to the family physician. Information on tests not discussed in this chapter can be obtained from commercial test suppliers, general reference books,[1] psychologists, or other trained professionals.

Table 13-1 lists those tests that are commonly used by family practice residency programs. The tests were identified through a survey in which questionnaires were sent to 337 of these programs.[2] Sixty percent of the contacted programs responded and approximately half reported that they taught and/or used psychological tests in their centers.

The most frequently used test, the Minnesota Multiphasic Personality Inventory or "MMPI," is also the most extensively studied test in the psychological literature. The MMPI contains 550 true-false questions concerned with a patient's health, habits, thoughts, moods, and opinions. Questions were selected on the basis of their empirically determined utility in differentiating psychiatric patients from a general reference population. Patient responses yield scores on ten clinical scales reflecting major clinical dimensions such as depression, anxiety, thought disorder, and hysteria. Validity scales also exist to identify individuals who tend to gloss over problems, malinger, or respond randomly to question items. Few tests make such detailed analyses of a patient's attitude toward self and the test.

The MMPI is suitable for patients aged 12 and over with sixth grade or better reading ability. It comes in individual booklet and card sort formats, or on recorded tapes for administration to disabled or illiterate patients. Administration of the test requires 60 to 90 minutes. An office receptionist, with only brief training, can give instructions for the test, and score test results in less than 10 minutes. Interpretation of the results can be provided by a psychologist, psychometrist, or one of a number of sourcebooks.[3, 4] Scoring and interpretation can also be obtained from one of several computer services.

Figure 13-1 provides an example of an MMPI test profile. The MMPI is useful in assessing levels of depression, anxiety, general distress, general personality characteristics, functional components contributing to physical illness and chronic pain. It also evaluates a patient's tendency to exaggerate, malinger, or gloss over problems. The MMPI is the classic example of an individually administered, objective personality inventory.

A different approach to the assessment of personality characteristics is the projective test. In general, this type of test is less useful to the family physician as it requires the assistance of a trained psychometrist and does not tend to yield quantifiable scores with acceptable reliability

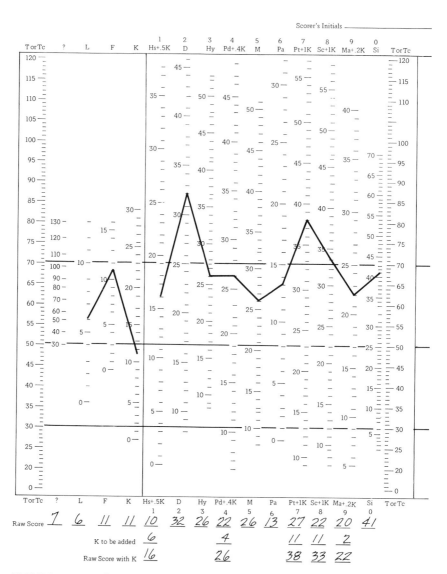

FIGURE 13-1.   The Minnesota Multiphasic Personality Inventory (MMPI).

and validity. However, one projective test used by the family practice residency programs surveyed was Rotter's Incomplete Sentence Blank. In this type of test the first words of a sentence are supplied (e.g., "My family is . . .") and the patient provides a concluding phrase. The patient is thereby allowed to project his own interpretation onto an open-ended stimulus. Interpretation of the results from this test is a more subjective task than using MMPI scale scores.

Two additional personality scales used with some frequency by family practice residency programs are the Zung and Beck depression scales. These scales are highly focused; concerned with a single attribute of a person's functioning. The scales are short objective instruments consisting of twenty questions or less. Forms are readily available from test publishers and even some drug companies. They provide norms for categorizing the level or severity of depression.[5, 6] Test results from short forms of this type can be used as screening devices, or to follow a patient's progress through treatment. Figure 13-2 reproduces the Zung Depression Scale.

A wide variety of tests have been developed for assessing an individual's level of intellectual functioning, and it is not surprising to find such tests being used by family physicians. However, the tests currently used in residency programs for assessing intellectual performance are time consuming and require specialized training to administer. These tests are the Wechsler Adult Intelligence Scale (WAIS) and the Wechsler Intelligence Scale for Children (WISC).

The last test used with any frequency in family practice residency programs is the Denver Developmental Screening Test. At first glance, this may not seem to be a psychological test as it is such a familiar tool in pediatric settings. Yet, the DDST does sample a set of patient behaviors in a standardized manner and provides normative data for comparing responses to healthy and ill individuals. These are the basic characteristics of a psychological test. The tasks on this test cover four major areas of development: personal-social, fine motor-adaptive, language, and gross motor. The test takes about ten to twenty minutes to administer and can be used for routine and periodic screening with children through age six.

CLINICAL APPLICATIONS OF PSYCHOLOGICAL TESTS

The family physician can use psychological tests in a similar manner to current use of laboratory tests. Tests that are simple, used often, and require limited specialized skills can be administered entirely in the physician's office—just as the hematocrit or gram stain is performed in the office laboratory. In other cases which require the skills of a psychome-

Name _____

Age _____ Sex _____ Date _____

	None OR a Little of the Time	Some of the Time	Good Part of the Time	Most OR All of the Time
1. I feel down-hearted, blue and sad				
2. Morning is when I feel the best				
3. I have crying spells or feel like it				
4. I have trouble sleeping through the night				
5. I eat as much as I used to				
6. I enjoy looking at, talking to and being with attractive women/men				
7. I notice that I am losing weight				
8. I have trouble with constipation				
9. My heart beats faster than usual				
10. I get tired for no reason				
11. My mind is as clear as it used to be				
12. I find it easy to do the things I used to				
13. I am restless and can't keep still				
14. I feel hopeful about the future				
15. I am more irritable than usual				
16. I find it easy to make decisions				
17. I feel that I am useful and needed				
18. My life is pretty full				
19. I feel that others would be better off if I were dead				
20. I still enjoy the things I used to do				

FiGURE 13-2. The Zung Depression Scale. © William W. K. Zung, 1965, 1974. All rights reserved.

194

trist or psychologist, the family physician will still ask specific questions and integrate test results into the patient's clinical management. This is analogous to the family physician's use of the diagnostic services of a radiologist or pathologist. In still other cases, decisions for psychological testing may be deferred to a psychologist as one would refer a patient for evaluation and management to a neurologist. In the survey of family practice residency programs described earlier, each of the above modalities were reportedly employed.

The decision to use a psychological test can be made for varied reasons. The physician may want to corroborate a clinical impression with the MMPI, assess the performance of a hyperactive child with the Denver Developmental Screening Test, document changes in a patient's mood through repeated administration of the Zung Depression Scale, or screen patients on some relevant behavioral dimension. In this manner tests can be used to corroborate clinical impressions, aid in differential diagnosis, objectively document patient status, or screen patients for particular characteristics. Additionally, psychological tests can be used as a self-assessment tool; physicians can compare their own impressions with the findings of a reliable and objective test instrument. Finally, psychological tests can be used as dependent measures in clinical outcome studies.

The choice of which test to use for a specific situation requires adequate understanding of the patient, the problem, the area of behavior to be measured, the available tests and their assets and limitations. Family physicians are most likely to employ psychological tests that can be administered to patients on an individual basis. Short test forms that patients complete on their own will prove most practical for administration in the physician's office. For reasons already discussed, physicians are also likely to find objective tests more useful than interpretive or projective psychometrics.

A number of psychological tests used in the surveyed residency programs do not meet the above criteria. For example, Rotter's Incomplete Sentence Blank is a projective type test relating to the concerns of psychiatrists or psychologists. The WAIS and WISC require specialized training and are cumbersome to administer. How can one account for the use of these tests by family physicians? The likely hypothesis is that when a question about testing arises, the family physician who is unfamiliar with psychometrics consults with a psychologist. Psychologists may not be so sensitive to the needs of family practice; they are likely to recommend those tests with which they are familiar. As a result, the current use of psychological tests by physicians may be shaped by the patterns of usage developed by psychologists, rather than formed by the needs of family practice.

Several scales exist that would seem particularly relevant to the interests and needs of family physicians. The Holmes-Rahe Life Stress Scale provides a convenient instrument for sampling changes in an individual's life, and weighting these events in terms of life stress units. Holmes and his associates have conducted studies that demonstrate a relationship between life-change units and physical illness.[7] A scale of similar utility has been developed by Jenkins to identify the Type A or coronary prone personality.[8] This type of scale can be used as a screening instrument in the family physician's office. Alternatively, it can be used with selected patients to document behavior patterns.

In contrast to the WAIS and WISC, there exist a number of short assessment instruments for evaluating intellectual functions. One example of such an instrument is the Shipley Institute of Living Scale, formerly called the Shipley-Hartford Retreat Scale. This individually administered paper and pencil test is presented on a single page with twenty vocabulary items and twenty abstraction items. The first five of each type of item are presented in Table 13-2. The items yield two scores called the Intellectual Quotient and the Conceptual Quotient; a low ratio of IQ to CQ suggests intellectual impairment of an organic nature. Age based norms are available for this test and raw scores can be converted to estimates of Wechsler's full scale scores.[9]

The Rotter Incomplete Sentence Blank is but one example of a general test format that may be of interest to family physicians. Rather than the sentence, "My family is . . .", the presurgical patient could complete

TABLE 13-2.   Sample Items from the Shipley Institute of Living Scale*

Vocabulary Items

1. TALK	draw	eat	speak	sleep
2. PERMIT	allow	sew	cut	drive
3. PARDON	forgive	pound	divide	tell
4. COUCH	pin	eraser	sofa	glass
5. REMEMBER	swim	recall	number	defy

Conceptual Items

1. 1 2 3 4 5 __
2. white black   short long   down __
3. AB   BC   CD   D __
4. Z Y X W V U __
5. 12321 23432 34543 456 __ __

* Reprinted with permission from The Institute of Living.

sentences like, "The thing I most fear is . . . ," or "I most want to. . . ." An example of a general self-description form is provided in Figure 13-3.[10] In time, family physicians may develop new formats that are highly relevant to their practice settings and to the problems of their patients.

Whenever a psychological test is administered, the results of that test should be discussed with the patient. When done in a thoughtful and constructive fashion, discussion of test results can open valuable areas for discussion. Based on test results, the physician can objectively present information and encourage the patient to cut down on stresses, develop relaxation skills, and redefine career objectives. One note of caution is needed when physicians assess the intellectual functioning of their patients. It is generally advised to not report specific IQ scores to patients as this may communicate to the individual a fixed level of functioning. This is unwarranted since cultural factors, the patient's attitudes toward testing, and motivational factors may have influenced the score obtained. In addition, professionals are well aware of the "slow" individual who with sufficient motivation makes tremendous gains in functioning. Reporting a fixed IQ score can have a demoralizing effect that is clinically unproductive and objectively unfounded.

Self-description:
Please complete the following:

I am _____
I am _____
I am _____
I am _____
I feel _____
I feel _____
I feel _____
I feel _____
I think _____
I think _____
I think _____
I think _____
I wish _____
I wish _____
I wish _____
I wish _____

FIGURE 13-3. **Incomplete Sentence Format for Self-Descriptions.***

* Reprinted from Lazarus AA: *Behavior Therapy and Beyond.* New York: McGraw-Hill, 1971, page 251.

CONCLUSIONS

Psychological tests offer a potential tool for the family physician. They can aid in the assessment of a wide number of behavioral issues, document patient status, screen for particular characteristics, and provide a gauge or standard against which the physician's own diagnostic skills can be compared. At the present time, the full application of psychological tests to family practice settings is yet to be realized. Patterns of test usage closely follow the patterns of usage developed by psychologists. The most useful psychological tests for medical settings remain to be identified. Indeed, family physicians may find it necessary to develop their own testing instruments based on clinical experience.

It is important to stress the limitations of psychological tests.[11] They are limited in their ability to make differential diagnoses without alternative and substantiating sources of data. Psychological tests are limited with regard to localization of brain lesions or other organic disease. General psychologicals are to be avoided; they often yield nothing more than nonspecific reports of varied test results.

The physician who uses psychological tests wisely will ask focused questions, for which specific tests have been designed. The physician will then use the results in conjunction with corroborating history, knowledge of the patient's self-reported problem, other laboratory findings, and awareness of the patient's attitude and approach to illness. As previously noted, test results can contribute to clinical judgment; they cannot replace it.

REFERENCES

1. Buros OK (ed): *Tests in Print*. Highland Park, New Jersey: Gryphon Press, 1974
2. Phillips WR, Rosen GM: Use of psychological tests in family practice residency programs. J Fam Prac 9:504–506, 1979
3. Dahlstrom WG, Welsh G, Dahlstrom L: *An MMPI Handbook: Volume I, Clinical Interpretation*. Minneapolis: University of Minnesota Press, 1972
4. Duckworth JC, Duckworth E: *MMPI Interpretation Manual for Counselors and Clinicians*. Muncie, Indiana: Accelerated Development, 1977
5. Zung WWK: A self-rating depression scale. Arch Gen Psychiatry 12:63–70, 1965
6. Beck AT, Beck RW: Screening depressed patients in family practice: A rapid technic. Postgrad Med J 52:81, 1972
7. Holmes TH, Masuda M: "Life Change and Illness Susceptibility." In BS Dohrenwend, BP Dohrenwend eds: *Stressful Life Events: Their Nature and Effects*. New York: John Wiley & Sons, 1974, pp. 45–72

8. Jenkins CD: Recent evidence supporting psychologic and social risk factors for coronary disease. N Eng J Med 294:987–994 & 1033–1038 (April 29 and May 6), 1976

9. Prado WM, Taub DV: Accurate prediction of individual intellectual functioning by the Shipley-Hartford. J Clin Psychol 22:294–296, 1966

10. Lazarus AA: *Behavior Therapy and Beyond.* New York: McGraw-Hill Book Company, 1971

11. Nathan PE: "Psychologic Testing." In P Solomon & VD Patch eds: *Handbook of Psychiatry,* 3rd ed. Los Altos, California: Lange Medical Publications, 1974

SECTION IV

Approaches to Treatment

CHAPTER 14

APPLICATIONS OF COUNSELING AND PSYCHOTHERAPY

G. GAYLE STEPHENS

Leston Havens wrote that the first great task of psychotherapy is to establish a relationship; the second is to bear what that relationship reveals.[1] The sober recognition of such responsible tasks ought to dissuade even the most cavalier among us from a dilettante attitude towards psychotherapy. At the same time such recognition ought not to intimidate the serious minded family physician from entering into therapeutic communication with patients. It is not feasible for family physicians to avoid doing some kind of psychotherapy; the question is, how self-conscious, deliberate, and responsible for it the physician will become.

DEFINITIONS

This chapter serves as an introduction to subsequent chapters which focus on special methods of psychological treatment for individuals, couples, and groups. The stage will be set for what follows by calling attention to some of the generic issues for psychotherapy in family practice.

First, there is the matter of definitions of terms. They should not overoccupy us, but it may be worthwhile to call attention to the three related terms of psychotherapy, counseling and patient education. It may not be possible to define these in a way that is completely satisfactory to all, but general characteristics can be stated. Patient education may be the simplest and clearest since it usually involves the transfer of information and knowledge from the physician to the patient. However, when attempting to deal with the patient's barriers to learning or resistance to adhering to a therapeutic regimen, the physician may find that attitudes, fears, family tradition, or cultural beliefs constitute the problem requiring a strategy going beyond the mere transfer of information.

Counseling may then become the proper term to describe the process by which attitudes and beliefs are recognized and explored in the interest of change. This should not mean, of course, that the physician simply tries to substitute his or her own beliefs for the patient's, or that the patient is attacked; but rather, that through the process of communication, the patient is assisted in examining attitudes and beliefs that may be inimical to health. Counseling may be preceded by a modifier, such as genetic, premarital, marriage, or sexual, indicating the focus of conversation. Counseling is also preferentially used to describe the activities of pastors, social workers, or counseling psychologists who may use that word as a psychiatrist might mean psychotherapy.

Psychotherapy can be used in a strict or in an extended sense. The former usually means that the theories and ideas of Freud or his followers are used as the conceptual basis for treatment; the latter may simply mean the use of any psychological measures to benefit the patient. Small listed over seventy techniques that qualify as psychotherapy[2]; while Levine, who also took the broader view, listed twenty-five methods for the general practitioner and fifteen others constituting advanced methods often requiring the services of a psychiatrist.[3]

Hollingshead and Redlich, whose classic study related the treatment of mental illness to the patient's social class, grouped psychiatrists into two dimensions, the analytic-psychologic (A and P) and the directive-organic (D and O).[4] The former "tend to wear street clothes in the office, come predominately (83 percent) from Jewish backgrounds, conduct longer and more frequent sessions with patients, and are generally introspective people believing in a psychologic etiology of mental illness." The D and O psychiatrists, mainly (75 percent) from Protestant backgrounds, give drugs, electric shock treatment, and advice. They wear white coats and read a completely different set of medical journals from the first group of psychiatrists. They do not use the couch and conduct physical examinations of their patients. Their therapy sessions are shorter and less frequent, and they hold the conviction that there is an organic etiology to most mental illness.[5]

The words dynamic, expressive, uncovering, and analytically-oriented are used for psychotherapies indebted for their theory to Freud. They do not use classical psychoanalytic methods such as the couch, five weekly sessions, and free association; but they do aim at broad change in the personality of the patient and accept the importance of early childhood experience, stages of personality development, unconscious motivation, and defense mechanisms.

Supportive psychotherapy is a derivative of analytic oriented therapy having a special relevance to general medicine and family practice. The goals of support are direct relief of symptoms and strengthening of the patient's defenses. Supportive psychotherapy focuses on conscious, current conflicts in reality. It is not aimed at insight, uncovering, or intensive interpretation. In contrast to classical psychoanalysis, the therapist is active, authoritative (not authoritarian), and demanding (limit setting).

Supportive psychotherapy is the basic tool of the family physician who is called upon to maintain long term relationships with many patients. At various times during the relationship the family physician may add a number of different techniques to supportive work but when completed the basic support remains. The rest of this chapter may be taken as a commentary on the characteristics of support in a family practice setting, while subsequent chapters describe some of the special techniques.

THE FAMILY PRACTICE SETTING

There are a number of constraints and advantages to the family practice setting that influence the nature of psychotherapy carried on there. Perhaps the most obvious constraints are the relatively large number of patients in a practice and the limited segments of time that can be spent with each. The patients also are unselected as to age, sex, or complaint so that each office day is unpredictable. The family physician must be able to shift focus from a well child, to a woman with abnormal vaginal bleeding or pelvic pain, to a geriatric patient complaining of weakness or aching joints. When a practice has become established, it is possible to better predict how much time certain patients will require; but control over the schedule is never complete. Furthermore, since most patients come to a family physician with a physical complaint, there is usually a lack of formal identification as to the occurrence of psychotherapy. In most instances the visit is accompanied by physical examination of a body part or an organ system, frequently terminating with a prescription or other attention to the patient's physical status.

There is also the very real problem to the family physician of adequate compensation for doing psychotherapy. The lack of formality in the schedule, along with the biases of medical insurance programs, mitigate against adequate identification and compensation for the family physician.

Finally, among the constraints is the lack of systematic thinking and teaching about psychotherapy in the family physician's education. There is general recognition of the importance of psychological and social factors in medical practice, but this often stops with exhortations to be more sensitive without supplying rigorous training in proper techniques. This lack may subvert the physician's confidence and lead them to undervalue services they provide.

Certain advantages counter the constraints to the family practice setting. First, the family physician may actually have more time to spend with a patient when the longitudinal dimension is taken into account. Once the data base has been acquired for a patient and a working relationship formed, the physician is free to establish the frequency and duration of future visits. Theoretically, the doctor-patient relationship can be maintained interminably with varying intensity. Second, the basic trust that is the foundation of every successful doctor-patient relationship is the best foundation for psychotherapy. The stigma the patient might feel with a psychiatrist does not exist in participating in a talking therapy with the family physician. Third, the family physician has access to multiple sources of information about the patient—the entire medical record, relatives, friends, and a social relationship that might exist between the patient and physician. This does not necessarily mean that the physician always seeks information from these sources, but in the normal course of events, knowledge comes to the observant and curious physician. Moreover, the family physician is one of the few professionals who has access to the patient's home. It is easy to arrange a home visit by the physician, a nurse, or social worker; there is no reason such visits cannot be initiated by the physician rather than by a request from the patient.

Finally, there are among the advantages of the setting three that should not be undervalued:

1. The lack of commitment to a single ideology of psychological treatment frees the physician to be eclectic and pragmatic. There can be shifts from ventilation and confession, life history discussion, or behavioral modification in the same patient at different points of life without violating one's vocational credentials or practice expectations.
2. There is the real probability that the costs of psychotherapy with a family physician will be less for the patient.
3. The family physician has permission to touch the patient. With proper respect, touching is an important element of the family physician's work.

Animal psychologists have equated mutual grooming behavior among primates with psychotherapy. If true, this suggests touching as therapy may belong to the deepest biological roots of the species. Touching is most often done in the course of physical examination when the site of a pain can be explored directly, in physical therapy and minor surgery; but it also occurs in a friendly handshake, a pat on the back, or a hand squeeze when taking leave of a bedfast patient at home or in the hospital. Patients come to associate relief, warmth, gentleness, and caring with the physician's hands; it is a diminished family physician who does not learn how to touch patients therapeutically.

HOW PSYCHOLOGICAL PROBLEMS ARE ENCOUNTERED IN FAMILY PRACTICE

Given the constraints and opportunities of the setting, how are psychological factors and problems identified in family practice? As already indicated, most patients present with a physical complaint, but there are characteristics of such complaints that increase the likelihood of finding underlying psychological factors. The following are six common conditions or circumstances often leading to the discovery of such factors.

1.   Complaints that in themselves are associated with a high frequency of psychological stress. Headaches are among the most common of these. Whether it be a muscle-contraction headache in the occipito-nuchal or frontal region; the classical one-sided, temporal throbbing of migraine; or the aching of sinus trouble, headache is a frequent sign of psychic stress or strain. Autonomic symptoms in general—light-headedness, dizziness, air hunger, dysphagia without obstruction, abdominal cramping, gaseous distention, alternating changes in bowel habits, urinary frequency, and hot or cold flashes—can all reflect an autonomic nervous system responding to stress.

2.   Vague and undifferentiated symptoms that may accompany depression. Fatigue, weakness, lack of energy, and loss of a sense of well-being are frequent motivations to seek medical care. When these are accompanied by mood changes, sleep disturbances, anorexia, constipation, and decrease in sexual activity, depression should be considered first; although there may be reasons why anemia, diabetes, hypothyroidism, and occult malignancy must be excluded by appropriate examinations.

3.   Other somatic complaints often associated with psychological factors are these:

1.   Pains or paresthesia that are anatomically or physiologically atypical.
2.   Complaints out of proportion to the degree of pathology identified.

3. Complaints not verified by physical, laboratory, or radiographic examinations.
4. Complaints persisting beyond a reasonable time for recovery from an acute illness, injury, or operation.
5. Dramatic but unexplained symptoms—episodes of loss of consciousness, paralysis, loss or change of vision, loss of voice, loss of bowel or bladder control, muscle spasms of large muscle groups.
6. Symptoms occurring under circumstances of possible secondary gain. Auto accidents, on-the-job injuries, injuries or illnesses due to the negligence of another person.

Of course, any of these could be due to specific diseases which the prudent physician will think about and exclude by appropriate examinations, but it is more likely that psychological factors will emerge if sought. The common mistake is to attribute the symptoms to a relatively minor or chronic disease that is discovered incidentally.

4. Patients often present with straight-forward psychological symptoms. Family physicians should become experts in recognizing these phenomena directly—even though the reasons for their presence may not be apparent. One of the straight-forward symptoms is anxiety. Anxiety is mediated through the sympathetic nerves and can be reproduced pharmacologically by epinephrine and its congeners. Hyperalertness, unexplained fear, restlessness, irritability, excitement, and insomnia represent central effects. The peripheral effects may involve the special-sense organs, skin, and the various visceral organ systems. Dry mouth, nasal congestion, flushing of the skin, and pupillary dilation are easily observable as are tachycardia, systolic hypertension, and hyperventilation. The patient may also report palpitations, dyspnea, chest pain or discomfort, choking or smothering sensation, dizziness, and paresthesia.

Anxiety may be chronic and persistent, or occur in attacks that may be so dramatic and frightening as to result in an emergency call or hospitalization. Such attacks can be produced by catecholamine secreting tumors, as in pheochromocytoma, or hyperthyroidism; but when they begin early in life (before age 40), are recurrent and not associated with marked physical exertion, life-threatening situations, or medical illness, anxiety disorders can safely be diagnosed. It is surprising how frequently the diagnosis of anxiety is overlooked by physicians and the patient is subjected to repeated and futile attempts to discover a disease. Such attempts are not only costly but are also risky; they often delay providing of the temporary relief of antianxiety drugs while psychological factors are being identified and managed.

Depression is a second symptom that should also be recognized on its own merits. Dysphoric mood changes are the hallmark. The patient feels sad, blue, despondent, discouraged, down in the dumps, all gone, and worried. Poor appetite, weight loss (ten pounds in a year or two pounds per week), insomnia, hypersomnia, loss of energy, loss of interest, difficulty in concentrating, guilt feelings, and thoughts of death complete the picture. The physician should determine when in the patient's life such symptoms began and whether or not they are recurrent, interspersed with manic or hypomanic states associated with losses, life changes, or physical illnesses. The identification of depression as a secondary phenomenon or as part of a primary affective disorder is important in management and prognosis.

The diagnosis of psychological symptoms can be assisted greatly by referring to an article written by Feighner et al.[6]

5.   Well-Person Examinations: It has been determined that about 20 percent of visits to family physicians are ostensibly well-person examinations—annual physicals, insurance and school examinations, preemployment physicals, and birth control surveillance. Many of these encounters involve a relatively hidden or sometimes secret motive; the patient actually has a health concern but is reluctant to express it until after it is determined whether or not it is safe to do so. The physician can conduct these examinations in such a way that the patient is given an opportunity to express such concerns. Sometimes a simple inquiry beginning with, "How do you feel about . . . getting more insurance, going to camp, going to college, and so forth" will open the door to the secret. The physician's knowledge of life stages, developmental tasks, and common, human reactions to change allows discreet, open-ended, gentle questioning that is not intrusive and often brings worrisome problems to light. The gentle, inquiring style of the physician can convert what might otherwise be a dull and routine part of practice into professionally gratifying experiences that are of immense benefit to patients.

6.   The patient's discovery of a new disease: This always calls for psychological sensitivity on the part of the physician. Disease represents a threat to the patient's bodily integrity and produces heightened awareness of vulnerability, disability, and death. It is a time for serious evaluation of one's habits, life style, occupation, and family relationships. It is a time of stress and crisis, full of fantasies about one's future, fears, guilt feelings, and anger. The physician should know that these things are occurring, even when the illness might not be all that serious from a strict medical perspective. This is an opportunity to assist patients work through their responses to illness, as well as evaluate other aspects of their lives that could profit from a constructive change.

It should be clear from this discussion that family physicians do not usually encounter psychological problems as clear cut, well-defined entities that are the primary reason for the patient's visit. Most often psychological problems are discovered in the course of routine medical work. It is possible for the physician to conduct an interview and examination in ways that either inhibit or facilitate such discovery. The beginning and the end of each visit are optimum times for such facilitation. In the first few minutes of each visit the physician can manifest openness so that the patient feels free to interject anything of concern, and be assured that it will be received as legitimate. At the end of each visit the physician can determine the patient's apparent satisfaction and allow time for questions. Many times the most important reasons for a visit will emerge at the end, often when the physician is ready to treat the next patient. This can be disconcerting and frustrating; but sensitive, experienced physicians learn to expect and value disclosures that are made. This does not imply that the physician can deal with psychological problems as afterthoughts; responding is largely a technical problem of learning how to reschedule the patient without causing offense.

SPECIFIC PSYCHOTHERAPEUTIC TASKS IN FAMILY PRACTICE

Given the unique characteristics of the family practice setting and the ways that psychological problems become manifest, there are a number of specific tasks that must be accomplished. These are recurrent and must be mastered over and over again. The family physician never gets beyond them. No matter how expert one becomes in medical practice, each patient is a new challenge to the physician's skills.

The importance of discovering the real reason for a patient's visit has already been pointed out. This has been described by Feinstein as the iatrotrophic stimulus, and it is not necessarily the same as the chief complaint or stated reason for the visit.[7] Identification of the iatrotrophic stimulus answers two questions: why this chief complaint and why now? It reflects the assumption that the patient has made a motivated decision to seek medical care and that circumstantial factors entered into that decision. Coming to see a doctor is not a casual incident in a patient's life; most people do not consult physicians often, although they have many episodes of ill health. How does an individual learn to define a problem as medical; and when is it bad enough to justify the time, expense, and possible discomfort of seeing a physician? We know that social and cultural factors affect this decision. Except in urgent or emergency situations when injury or pain is the overriding and compelling factor, most symptoms exist for a period of time before they are recognized by the patient. Some patients are stoical and ignore symptoms until they become intolerable. Usually they let someone else know as a way of gaining perspective. If the other person concurs that the symptom is important, a step has been taken towards the doctor. Sometimes it is a family decision; at other times the illness or death of a friend, relative, or fellow employee activates a person to become a patient. Rarely does anyone come to a physician without having ideas of what might be the trouble. Balint called this process "organizing the illness." It is a wise physician who can discover the way an illness has been organized prior to the consultation, as well as discovering the iatrotrophic stimulus.[8]

One may not always be able to discover the iatrotrophic stimulus on the first visit. It certainly can not be demanded, but it should always have a high priority on the physician's agenda.

Patient example

A 65-year-old woman consulted a physician for a cancer checkup by which she meant a pap smear, and a breast and pelvic examination. She was excessively concerned to reassure him that this was simply routine and that she had no complaints. It was only after the examination was completed, the patient had dressed and the physician was about ready to terminate the visit that in response to his open-ended inquiry, "Tell me about your habits," the patient confessed that she had been taking amphetamine diet pills for five years and was worried that they might be harming her. She assumed that normal findings on a check up would mean that the pills were safe.

A second task for the physician is to develop the professional capacity to conceal surprise at what the patient might confide. This skill can be acquired early if it is recognized as important. Patients often have fantasies about how risky it is to share their secrets with the physician. They imagine shock at their confession of masturbation, or that the physician will think them terrible that sometimes they wish their children dead, or that they will be rejected if they tell about their dreams of homosexuality. The physician's reaction to secret information is often expressed nonverbally by facial movements, gestures, an embarrassed silence, or hasty and lame reassurance. The patient is comforted by a lack of surprise and a facilitative response allowing further elaboration of the story.

Patient example

A young mother began by saying, "I know you are going to think I am a terrible mother, but I've got to tell somebody. Twice in the past week I've had a horrible dream that I poured scalding water on my baby. Doctor, am I a terrible mother?" After a short silence the physician replied, "Do you think you are a terrible mother?" She said, "No, but why would I have a dream like that?" Then she continued her account.

A third task is acquiring the ability to translate the patient's metaphors. Most patients use metaphors since they lack a medical vocabulary to express their symptoms. Some of these are humorous, some are pathetic, but all are serious and important. Doctors tend to react to the patient's language in terms of its degree of concreteness. Some patients can only complain of pain; and when the pain is bizarre, the language theatrical, the location nonanatomical, and the pattern unphysiological, the physician is frustrated by the inappropriate description. Pauline Bart wrote of the "vocabularies of distress," and reported a study showing that patients who use concrete language most often get treated somatically—even surgically if they keep complaining.[9]

Patient example

A student came to the Student Health Clinic three times within a month requesting a VD test. On the first two occasions he was examined and a blood sample was drawn. On the third visit the physician, on a hunch said, "There is a question I'd like to ask you, but I don't know how." The student replied, "Do you mean, am I gay?" An account followed of a long-standing homosexual relationship that was ending. The student was using the VD test as a sexual and medical metaphor to obtain medical attention in the hope that his problem would be discovered.

Closely akin to the task of perceiving and translating metaphors of illness, is the unending task of cultivating one's self-awareness in the interest of diminishing biases and idiosyncracies. Though all physicians strive for scientific objectivity in clinical decisions, they practice with a personal style reflecting their own history, social class, and personality characteristics. Balint termed this style "apostolic function," and it determines the unique characteristics of each physician's practice and qualifies relationships with individual patients.[10] It often determines what types of patients become incorporated into the practice and even with what frequency certain diagnoses are made. Patients who might be regarded with special interest or fascination by one physician might be considered hopeless neurotics by a colleague.

Certain patient characteristics constitute problems for most physicians, e.g., gross obesity, negligent or noncompliant behavior. However, more subtle problems are created by the physician's sense of integrity, attitude toward pain and suffering, social consciousness, sense of fair play, and honor. Sometimes these affect clinical judgments more than is recognized.

Patient example

A resident physician was asked by his attending physician to meet a patient in the emergency ward. The resident had to wait thirty minutes before the patient arrived. The patient turned out to be a grossly obese woman with poor personal hygiene whose complaints the resident thought were exaggerated. Moreover, the family members who accompanied the patient seemed to want to dump her into the hospital. Irritated by the delay, offended by the patient's person and morally indignant at the family, the resident missed the diagnosis of congestive heart failure; not because he did not know the pathophysiology and clinical signs and symptoms of heart failure, but because his judgment was impaired by his personal characteristics in that particular encounter. The patient was admitted by her attending physician and lost thirty pounds of edema fluid during the first week of treatment.

Unfortunately, it is possible for the physician to complete medical school without having to subject his or her biases, prejudices and personality to critical supervision. Yet, this task is essential for learning effective psychotherapy. Psychiatrists refer to the physician's unconscious and symbolic reactions to a patient as countertransference. The patient's similar unconscious and symbolic reactions to the doctor are referred to as transference. One does not have to be a psychiatrist to become involved in transference-countertransference interactions. They occur in every continuing doctor-patient relationship, and may be more important in determining the ultimate quality of patient care than the physician's factual knowledge and technical skills. The surest way to learn about these interactions is to have one's clinical work supervised by psychologically sensitive and expert teachers and peers. It is a specific task.

The final tasks discussed here are the ability to raise the patient's consciousness and acceptance of psychological factors, and the preparation of the patient for consultation and/or referral to a psychotherapist. A great deal of a family physician's most effective work occurs in these tasks.

A patient's initial reaction to the suggestion that psychological factors are significant in an illness, or that consultation with a psychiatrist is recommended, is likely to be negative. Patients may think of such information as rejection, blame, or as preposterous, and they may resort to a number of tactics to counter the idea. "You mean this is all in my head!" or "You think I'm crazy!" are statements that may be heard scores of times in a physician's practice life-time. This is especially true when the suggestion of psychogenic factors comes at the end of a long and futile search for organic disease. The physician's own sanity may be called into question by a belligerent patient; or the patient may more subtly appeal to the physician's feeling of omnipotence by saying, "But, Doctor, you are the only one who understands me," or "But, Doctor, you are the only one who can help me."

Planning a strategy to avoid these sometimes tense and uncomfortable impasses should begin very early in a patient's care. Rather than thinking in terms of either psychological or organic conditions, the physician should cultivate the discipline of considering both at the outset. This is done by including both issues in taking the patient's history. One can move back and forth between these domains in the interviews; there are a number of nodal points when it is easy to shift the focus to the psychological domain without provoking the patient's resistance—or by provoking it gently. When developing the history of the present illness one might say, "What are the circumstances under which symptom X is likely to occur?", "What effects has this illness (or these symptoms) had on your daily life?", "What feelings have you had about the fact that these symptoms are occurring?", or "What thoughts have you had about what might be causing these symptoms?" Even if one does not receive psychological answers to these questions, the idea of including them has been introduced at an early stage. The start of the system review is another opportune nodal point. One might say, "Tell me about your general health," "How is your strength (energy, sense of well-being)?", or "Do you consider yourself a healthy person?" Any question that invites the patient to reflect on his or her general health is likely to be revealing.

Gentle probing and open-ended inquiries about the family, personal, and social histories are ideal occasions to gain a clear view of the patient's current situation. What housing is the patient living in? Who else lives there now? Any recent changes? One can usually raise the question of mood or disposition without seeming to depart from the medical model. "Have there been any recent changes in your life?" is an especially cogent question and may be followed by, "Are you expecting any changes in the near future?"

Finally, the physical examination is an appropriate occasion to continue the psychosomatic dialogue. Questions that may have been forgotten or purposefully omitted during the present illness and system review can be phrased as each organ system is examined. Inquiring about either surgical or traumatic scars is especially helpful in reminding the patient of forgotten incidents that often have an associated story. The writer has found that examination of the genitalia is a natural time to begin the sexual history. "Have you had any problem with your sexual organs?" is a simple lead-in to questions about specific functions, erection, impotence, orgasm, satisfaction, recent changes in function, and venereal diseases.

This style of medical interviewing should tie together in the mind of both participants the inextricable relatedness of psychological and organic functions. It leads quite naturally to a similar diagnostic and management strategy. When laboratory or radiographic studies are indicated, it is helpful for the physician to indicate the nature of the information desired and to even predict the probable results. In this way the physician averts a future encounter when a series of expensive but normal laboratory or radiographic studies are reported to the patient who then replies, "Well if all these tests are normal, then what's causing my (symptom)?" This is a poor time to introduce the notion of psychological factors, and patients will be justifiably irritated by such an approach. It is much better to be able to say, "As we expected your tests do not indicate the presence of diseases X, Y, or Z; and as we discussed at your previous visit, perhaps we should give further consideration to certain things that are going on in your life." Even if the patient replies, "Yes, but . . ." there has been a previous discussion, and judgments on how to proceed can then be made.

CONCLUSIONS

Family physicians should not be doctrinaire, dogmatic, or sectarian in their work. They should be able to adapt and utilize information from a variety of sources and disciplines. There is no easy shortcut to a bag of tricks and techniques that eliminate the risk, effort, and cost of intimate involvement in the lives of our patients. It is tempting to suppose that by relying on the biology and technology of medicine we can evade the need to deal with the human reactions of our patients, or leave those reactions to somebody else. Too often there is nobody else. Physicians can learn and cultivate a psychological sensitivity to the feelings and behavior of patients. This is not so much a function of time as it is of intent and attention. A ten-minute encounter can be as sensitive as an hour if we have the will to make it so. Once we have identified and estimated the intensity of emotional, social, and cultural factors, we can make a second-level decision about management. We may choose to manage the problem ourselves, and devise a plan as specific as anything else we do; or we can seek assistance through consultation or referral. The decision to refer also requires the knowledge of what and who is available, what methods and orientation they utilize, and what the indications are for a particular type of problem. In every case we should not underestimate the long-term value of a proper supportive relationship between our patient and ourselves.

REFERENCES

1. Havens L: Anatomy of suicide. N Eng J Med 272:401–408, 1965
2. Small L: *The Briefer Psychotherapies.* New York: Brunner/Mazel Pub., 1971
3. Levine M: *Psychotherapy in Medical Practice,* 18th ed. New York: The Macmillan Co., 1942, 1966
4. Hollingshead AB, Redlich FC: *Social Class and Mental Illness.* New York: Wiley, 1958
5. Chessick RD: *Technique and Practice of Intensive Psychotherapy.* New York: Jason Aronson, Inc., 1974
6. Feighner JP, Robins E, et al: Diagnostic criteria for use in psychiatric research. Arch Gen Psychiatry 26:57–63, 1972
7. Feinstein A: *Clinical Judgment.* Baltimore: Williams and Wilkins Co., 1967
8. Balint M: *The Doctor, His Patient and the Illness.* New York: International Univ. Press, Inc., 1957, p. 2
9. Bart PB: Social structure and vocabularies of discomfort. J Health and Social Behavior, 9:188–193, 1968
10. Balint, ibid.

CHAPTER 15

CRISIS INTERVENTION

RICHARD M. YARVIS AND BILL D. BURR

This chapter will present concepts and practices relating to a set of techniques which have come to be known as crisis intervention. Before doing so, it is necessary to define the term crisis and to illustrate some of the more common crises that people experience. It will also be necessary to discuss some fundamental principles that have evolved from etiological theories of crisis formation. This chapter will describe how crises are likely to present to the primary care physician and those sign posts which are important for recognizing patients in crisis. The process of crisis intervention will be described, and available data relating to the efficacy of crisis intervention will be considered.

DEFINITION OF CRISIS

Physicians who often assess human beings from a physiological perspective view them as being either in or out of a state of homeostatic balance. The principle of homeostasis can be applied as well to the psychological status of people. From a psychological point of view, crisis theorists such as Smith,[1] Caplan,[2] and Rapoport[3] have suggested that under some circumstances human beings may be considered to be in psychological homeostatis, but in other circumstances an imbalance or disequilibrium can occur. When in homeostatic balance people confront and master the various tasks and problems of living that commonly afflict all lives. These tasks include the successful mastery of internal stimuli, our fears and insecurities, as well as mastery of external stimuli comprising the usual and unusual stresses of life. Under most circumstances people are able to manage, cope, or master such stresses without significant outside assistance. Occasionally, they may feel overwhelmed by their feelings or by circumstances, but they usually recover quickly and find solutions to problems independently.

A number of circumstances can impinge upon an individual to affect this steady state of adequate coping. The stimuli or stress can be overwhelming in intensity. A feeling, impulse, or thought can have such intensity that even a normal individual with average coping skills cannot manage it adequately. Similarly, some external stressful life-event can be of such intensity, and so traumatic that a person who ordinarily copes well with stress is overwhelmed.

Patient Example 1

A young, married man in his early 20s with a small child has led a successful and happy married life. He works in the publishing industry and, while not altogether happy with his work, he is reasonably successful at it. He has friends and interests and has been coping quite well. Suddenly he finds himself at night with the urge to stab his small child and his wife. The thought recurs almost every night. The young man is badly frightened by his urge which he describes as quite powerful, still resistible, but becoming stronger. He becomes increasingly anxious and depressed, not knowing quite how to handle his impulses. He insists that he loves both his child and his wife and would not want to see them come to any harm. As the urge grows in intensity, he becomes increasingly more anxious and feels less and less able to cope. Here is an example of an internal stimulus causing stress and precipitating a crisis.

Patient Example 2

An unmarried woman in her early thirties with a successful career in interior design leads a happy, outgoing, and active social life. She has many friends and appears to be coping interpersonally and professionally in a superior manner. Suddenly she is assaulted in the middle of the night by a stranger who has broken into her apartment. She reports the assault to the police, obtains medical assistance, and finds that she has sustained no serious organic damage. The woman increasingly experiences more and more anxiety and depression, and unaccountably feels guilty. She becomes fearful of leaving her home, her active and social life deteriorate rapidly and within a matter of weeks she begins to lead a lonely, isolated, and frightened existence. Here an overwhelming external trauma has precipitated a crisis.

Stresses need not be unusual in their intensity to produce crises, instead a person's capacity to cope with stresses that do not exceed ordinary bounds can be impaired temporarily or permanently. Such individuals are especially vulnerable to stress and to the disequilibrium which it can cause. The impairment of coping skills may be due to illness, fatigue, the effects of medication, and other causes. Physicians should be aware that medical illnesses or treatments (e.g., cancer chemotherapy) can weaken coping skills and produce special vulnerabilities in patients.

Patient Example 3

A 55-year-old business man with a wife and three married children has always been able to aggressively manage both his personal and professional affairs. He is seen by his peers, his friends, and his family as an active, forceful, and decisive individual who can make decisions and cope with anything. Suddenly the man's business partner must retire. During an interim period while a replacement is being sought, this man must work 15 to 18 hours a day trying to do the job of both partners. He gets little sleep, eats irregularly, and gets progressively less recreation time. After several months, business stresses that he could previously cope with become unmanageable. He becomes listless and indecisive. His previous sensitivity for the feelings of other people diminishes and he becomes irritable, irascible, and tense. Moreover, he becomes depressed. In this example, a man whose ego strengths have been drained begins to lose his capacity to cope with stresses that he previously managed quite well.

These three vignettes illustrate some major possibilities which alone or together may create the circumstances in which a crisis can occur. Exposure to some stressful event generated from within or without, and the individual's capacity to cope when stress occurs, produce the potential for the development of a crisis.

STRESSFUL LIFE EVENTS AND CRISES

Some workers in the field of crisis theory, such as Bloom,[4] and Parad and Caplan[5] have stressed the concept of a precipitating stress being invariably associated with the development of crises. Parad has even suggested that calculation of the probability of a crisis occurring can be based on three factors: (1) the probability that the stressful event will occur; (2) the probability that a given individual will be exposed to such a stress; and (3) the vulnerability of that individual to the stress.

Turning to the work of Gerald Caplan,[6] we find another useful principle to distinguish between kinds of stresses. Caplan describes both developmental and accidental stresses. The former are normal components of the maturational development of individuals; they are ubiquitous in life. These are the stresses of growth and development, such as separation in childhood, marriage, and parenthood. On the other hand, accidental crises are not normal stresses. Such calamities as illness, injury, business reversal, the loss of a loved one, and others fall into this category.

Two major views concerning the importance of such stresses have been debated by investigators over the past 10 years. According to one view articulated most clearly by Holmes and Rahe,[7] any change or readjustment regardless of its meaning to the individual is stressful and may precipitate a crisis. Thus, it is change and the necessity of readjustment that are critical, not a particular characteristic of the stress. Developmental and accidental stresses are equally likely to precipitate a crisis. The second view of stress and its relationship to crises has been articulated by a number of writers including Paykel,[8] Myers,[9] Brown and Birley.[10] They suggest that it is not readjustment or change per se, but the necessity of coping with undesirable or threatening change that is critical in the development of crises. This view of stressful life events is more complicated than the first view, since under varying circumstances stresses will be considered positive or negative. A young, unmarried woman just starting out in a career who becomes pregnant may consider pregnancy as an undesirable event. The same woman, married and eager to have children, might consider the pregnancy as very desirable and hence, not stressful. In both cases the pregnancy will involve change and readjustment. Recent data examining these two views of change suggest that undesirable or threatening change rather than change per se is much more likely to precipitate crisis.[11, 12] If this view continues to prove correct, accidental stresses should prove more likely to precipitate crises than developmental stresses.

To summarize, a crisis is a disruption in the psychological equilibrium of an individual such that the capacity to cope with one or more parameters of life is significantly impaired. At such times, individuals cannot master problems that they otherwise might be capable of mastering. Alternately, the particular problem's magnitude may be so great that it defies the coping skills of a normally adequate ego. By definition, crises are time-limited and the term "crisis" should not be used to define a chronic condition in which coping is impaired. Crises are usually responses to some overt, demonstrable, and readily defined stress situation. Less frequently, an obvious precipitating stress is not readily apparent.

Both the healthy and the mentally ill may experience crises. In fact, mentally ill individuals may have less ego strength resulting in greater vulnerability to stress and to crises; but crises are experienced by many persons who are not afflicted by mental illness.

The resolution of a crisis is usually defined as a return to a precrisis level. When navigated successfully, a crisis can add to a person's repertoire of problem-solving skills. Crises which are not resolved successfully can lead to a lower level of function.

THE STAGES OF CRISIS

A crisis is by definition time-limited. Most investigators define the characteristic duration of a crisis as between several days and 6 to 8 weeks in length.[13] The state of crisis can be characterized as evolving through four stages. In stage one the stressful event precipitates a disequilibrium. The disequilibrium is characterized by a mild sense of tension or anxiety as a problem in need of solution is perceived.

The onset of stage two is characterized by the application of normal problem solving techniques and the recognition of their inadequacies. The initial mild anxiety now builds. The problem becomes a preoccupation to which all available coping skills are concentrated. Stage two may last several days. If coping skills are successful, the crisis aborts. If not, the process goes on to stage three.

Stage three is characterized by ever increasing tension and confusion. Added to this is a state of mild to moderate depression, frustration, and feelings of futility. A sense of panic may set in. Functioning deteriorates rapidly in many spheres and withdrawal begins. These phenomena are a consequence of the introduction of emergency coping techniques turned to out of a sense of desperation. At this point, individuals may ask for help from friends, family members, or even professionals. Stage three may last for weeks. If the emergency steps undertaken in stage three are not successful or if assistance is not obtained, the process proceeds to stage four.

In stage four anxiety and depression become intolerable. The individual now takes defensive actions by adopting either maladaptive or socially unacceptable behavior, or by developing symptomatic illness. The development of symptoms constitutes a way to bind anxiety, thereby reducing free-floating anxiety. Maladaptive behavior and symptomatic mental illness provide relief from manifest anxiety, but the risk of community sanctions or ego dysfunction is considerable.

There are several warnings for spotting and aborting the progression of a crisis state. A key factor to look out for is change in the patient's characteristic behavior. Affectual change, such as the patient who suddenly becomes anxious or depressed, can be a telltale sign. Patients who fall into this category suddenly experience vague physical symptoms with no organic cause for which they seek medical attention. Sudden change in functional status, such as impairments of school or work performance may be indicative of crisis. Patients who suddenly begin making demands on their physicians for time and attention unaccompanied by specific and concrete medical illness should be assessed for the possibility that the patient is in crisis. In such a case, the patient is attempting to enlist the primary care physician as a resource to assist him in coping. Any patient who has suffered significant stress should be observed for a developing crisis. Thus, the patient who has come to see the primary care physician and parenthetically mentions a forthcoming retirement, or the imminent prospect of children leaving the nest may be on the verge of a crisis. Any serious illness or injury may precipitate a crisis. In such cases, other family members should be remembered for they also may be experiencing crisis precipitating stress. In summary, the physician must be wary of sudden or uncharacteristic change in a patient's emotional, physical, or behavioral status. Additionally, the physician should be alert to the occurrence of stress, especially stress with negative connotations.

CASE ILLUSTRATIONS OF CRISES

Physicians should remember that routine injuries or illnesses are anything but routine to a patient; they may constitute the precursor of a crisis. Moreover, a patient's coping skills may be impaired or overwhelmed during illness episodes. Support in the way of reassurance, adequate information about the nature of the illness and its treatment, and a demonstration of competence on the part of the physician can go a long way toward augmenting the patient's coping skills.

Case Illustration

A 51-year-old white male has been admitted to a hospital with chest pain and is in mild congestive heart failure. His condition is stabilized and subsequent diagnostic workup reveals occlusion of a major coronary vessel. Corrective surgery is advised. In spite of sedating medications, the patient becomes increasingly agitated, tense, and finally irrational. After surgery is performed, the patient becomes manifestly paranoid and believes that the nursing staff is trying to poison him. In a period of less than three days, this patient's condition has deteriorated from a condition which can be characterized as a state of mild anxiety to one of a paranoid psychosis. After this patient had become overtly paranoid, a psychiatric consultation was requested. A combination of psychotropic medication, reassurance, and information about prognosis alleviated the patient's psychiatric condition which improved within 48 hours.

The above case vignette is not uncommon. It is quite possible that this chain of events could have been initially avoided. The patient was never prepared adequately for surgery. The stress of major surgery was added to that of his initial illness. Although the patient was in competent hands, he never received sufficient reassurance. An added lack of critical information increased his anxiety, and when this was neither recognized nor dealt with by the staff, a crisis resulted. In this weakened state, the patient's own coping mechanisms failed and overt mental illness developed.

Developmental stresses more often lead to crises if they come at the wrong time, are heaped upon other current stresses, or touch upon some particular vulnerability of the individual. Separation experiences, marriage, and the birth of children are all stressful developmental events which can precipitate crises. Below is an example of such a reaction.

Case Illustration

An 18-year-old female college freshman was brought to a crisis clinic by her family after they had unsuccessfully tried to help with psychotic behavior of several days' duration. No prior history of any emotional disability was reported. During a series of six meetings, the family with the aid of the therapist, began to wrestle with the following issues: (1) the departure from the home for college of the last child (the patient); (2) the mother's mounting fears of future purposelessness in her own life; (3) the patient's concurrent struggle with emancipation from home and concern about her mother's apparent and mounting depression; and (4) the father's relative isolation from the unfolding family disequilibrium. The patient began to examine her ambivalence and guilt over leaving home, and her sense of responsibility for her mother's depression. As she did this, her psychotic symptoms disappeared. After six sessions, the family was discharged from the clinic. At the patient's request, she was referred for further ambulatory psychotherapy.

It is likely that intervention and assistance would have been helpful at an earlier point in this case. Unfortunately, neither the girl's own internal resources, nor her home environment was sufficiently helpful to avert a crisis and the resulting psychosis. A therapist often must look beyond the identified patient and deal with the problems of other family members.

Stresses resulting from interpersonal or family relationships also can precipitate crises. The man or woman suddenly announcing to an unsuspecting mate a wish for a separation or divorce can cause a family crisis. In families with communication difficulties, children who act out by truancy, drug abuse, or sexual promiscuity can precipitate a crisis. The example below illustrates one such example.

Case Illustration

A 16-year-old high school student is noted by her parents to be mildly depressed, uncharacteristically irritable, and withdrawn. She is usually outgoing, happy, and energetic. The parent-child relationship has been good in the past; the parents initially take a supportive posture, and remain available for communication. The parents also employ some mild confrontation about the rapid and definite change from their daughter's normal behavior pattern. For a while, the girl's manifest irritability and growing anxiety increases. Then suddenly she breaks down in tears and explains that she has recently found out that she is pregnant. The parents are initially shocked and angry, but subsequently are able to show considerable sensitivity and support. A series of discussions follows within the family, then between the daughter and the family physician. As soon as she is aware that her parents will not abandon her, and will be supportive and helpful, the girl's anxiety and irritability diminish. An abortion is finally decided upon. Both parents accompany her to the doctor where the procedure is carefully and thoroughly explained. The girl experiences some anxiety and guilt, but she is able to discuss her feelings.

In this example, a crisis has been averted because of good parent-child communication. Sufficient time has been taken to explore all relevant issues. If these steps had not been taken, the probable result would have been either psychiatric symptomatology or some sort of dissocial behavior.

Unemployment, occupation- or school-related stresses can precipitate crises. Retirements are rarely planned well, therefore they can cause significant trauma and precipitate crises. Poor school performance, or the failure to achieve some education-related objective can become a significant source of stress, and in some instances can precipitate crises.

Case Illustration

A young man in his last year of college has applied for admission to five medical schools. He had made this career choice in the middle of high school. His parents endorse and place a premium on this educational objective, and are encouraging him to pursue it. He perceives this encouragement as a manifestation of the importance they place on his becoming a physician. He has done moderately well in college, and has some expectation of achieving his objective. By late spring of his senior year, he has not been accepted by any of the medical schools to which he has applied. He has been rejected outright by three of the schools, and is on the waiting list of three others. He begins to make frantic phone calls to other schools and to the schools on whose waiting lists he has been placed. These calls have a sense of panic about them, and when the schools cannot reassure him, his anxiety builds. In desperation he turns for advice to a family friend, a business associate of his father. This man is seen by the young man as a stable, interested adult. The man helps him to understand that he has mistaken his parents' support for parental pressure. Moreover, he helps the young man realize that his parents' opinion of him will not change as a consequence of nonadmission to medical school. This recognition helps him to significantly reduce his anxiety and he begins to explore alternative plans, should medical school admission not be forthcoming.

In this example, the young man's own coping skills suffice with only minimal assistance from another person. In some instances individuals can, after a short period of anxiety and disorganization, stabilize matters for themselves. Intervention before an individual has attempted to master a situation can be as ill-advised as too little intervention given too late. Thus, the intervenor always walks a tightrope. One must intervene just enough and just soon enough to provide help that is really needed. In the previous example, the support of an older and respected individual augmented the self-mastery process just enough to help the individual gain a realistic appraisal of the situation.

Death or the anticipation of death are serious and significant stresses which can precipitate crises. These crises may occur in the dying, or in the family members of the dead or dying.

Case Illustration

A man in his mid-30s, married and the father of two young children, seeks out the advice and support of his family's physician. The man's wife has cancer and is likely to die within a few months. He is clearly overwhelmed, and needs help and support to deal with all the problems attendant upon his catastrophe. The man exhibits evidence of both depression and anxiety. He is unsure of how to cope with his wife, his children, and his own sense of impending loss. How and whether to tell his wife the seriousness of her illness (she has not yet been told), and how to prepare the children for the impending loss of their mother are problems which must be dealt with. The physician is able to help to prepare the wife. He also arranges for several visits with a child psychiatrist to help the man deal appropriately with his children. Both physicians provide support and a genuine concern for the man's anguish. Other family members are mobilized to provide support as well.

Crises are sometimes precipitated by the onset of mental illness in a family member. Psychoses are especially apt to do this because of the extreme severity of their manifestations, and because the behavior associated with them is so difficult to understand.

Case Illustration

The parents of a 17-year-old girl present at the crisis clinic of a local hospital. The daughter has many of the classical signs of schizophrenia. Her reality testing is grossly impaired, she has a thought disorder, and her affect is flattened and inappropriate. She rambles on and on in a nonsensical manner. She is clearly frightened, and exhibits the signs of depersonalization and derealization. Her parents are very anxious, since they cannot understand what is happening. All three look drained and on the brink of major personal and family disorganization. If a family crisis is to be averted, several steps must be taken. First, the girl must receive immediate treatment. This will include the use of major tranquilizers. Second, the parents will require assistance. They must be educated about the nature of schizophrenia and what can be done about it. Moreover, they must be helped through the current episode with advice about how to deal with the patient. They should be enlisted to assist in the treatment process as well.

If all of the above measures are taken, then illnesses can be faced by families without major family disorganization.

There is one additional precipitator of crises that should be discussed briefly, and which is fundamentally different from the examples discussed above. This is the natural disaster. Natural disasters such as floods, hurricanes, earthquakes, or massive accidents undermine the capacity of the victim to cope. They wreak death and injury upon communities, and they disrupt normally present support systems. Such catastrophes are as likely to produce significant emotional damage as they do physical damage. Yet, because emotional damage is often unrecognized, it goes untreated. Crisis intervention should be as active a part of disaster as is intervention for physical trauma. Crisis teams ought to be mobilized along with all other medical and human service teams when disaster strikes.

THE NATURE AND EFFECTIVENESS OF CRISIS INTERVENTION

Persons experiencing crises sometimes require the assistance of external resources to assist in the resolution of their difficulties. Such external resources can augment the coping skills of the individual and mobilize family resources. Such resources also can provide direct assistance in the form of crisis intervention. Crisis intervention is a set of techniques developed in medical and nonmedical settings. These techniques have been designed specifically to deal with crises, rather than more chronic difficulties. This section examines the characteristics of crisis intervention, and explains how the techniques work. The reader is also referred to the particularly good work of Langsley[14] and Parad.[15]

Crisis intervention is time-limited and constitutes a form of brief intervention. Crisis intervention, if successful at all, is likely to accomplish its aim within 4 to 6 weeks. The number of interventions that actually take place during that period is variable and will depend upon the clinical needs of the specific case. Interventions may be limited to a single session or to as many as twelve to fifteen sessions. Most commonly eight to ten sessions suffice. A time-limited contract for services should be made with the patient.

Once a case is undertaken, the patient should have rapid and ready accessibility to the crisis intervenors, any time of the day or night. Once a crisis situation has been stabilized, the need for interventions outside of scheduled sessions will be relatively rare. In fact, once patients know that help is available at any hour of the day or night, they are reassured and rarely make use of it.

Crisis intervention is current-situation and current-problem oriented. It cannot and should not attempt to help people resolve long-standing problems. This is not to say that the intervenor should not learn about the patient's past life and long-standing problems that may contribute to the crisis, but the focus must be on the current problem; the problem that precipitated the patient's state of panic. The primary care physician will play varying roles in this process. The physician may simply act as a source of referral, or may become an active source of support. To be better prepared for the latter role, physicians should give serious consideration to continuing medical education courses that teach the techniques of crisis intervention.

Crisis intervention acts to mobilize coping skills in the patient, and in his or her family. Patients and their families are encouraged and assisted to find solutions for the current problems. To do this, the intervenor must support, comfort, and interpret. The intervenor must clarify communication problems in families, and must improve upon communication skills.

Crisis intervention must actively explore the precipitating stresses that led to the crisis. When such information is not spontaneously brought to the attention of the crisis intervenor, the physician must search for it. The identification of precipitants enables the intervenor and the person in crisis to identify a starting point from which to deal with the current problem.

Crisis intervention is a process in which the patient and, when necessary, the family participate very actively. In this type of intervention the patient cannot sit back and wait to be helped. The therapist, the patient, and the patient's family work together in a most active type of collaboration to define the current problem and devise a series of steps that will lead to a solution. A therapist's own solutions that are not arrived at jointly with patients will rarely alleviate a crisis. Crisis intervenors can augment the problem solving skills of patients, but they cannot supplant those skills.

Crisis intervention should involve the patient's family whenever possible. Families have much to contribute. They know the patient. They have the time, energy, and concern which will support the patient through a critical period. Physicians who have less time, but more objectivity, can be a superb bridge between the patient and other family members.

Crisis intervention will only be facilitative if patients are not overwhelmed by anxiety, depression, or guilt. Where psychoactive drugs can be helpful in alleviating such painful feeling states, they should be used without hesitation. Patients, and even families, who have been sleepless for nights should be medicated appropriately so that they can rest and reconstitute their strength.

Crisis intervention requires adequate information about the patient's past and current life, but this information must be collected in a minimum of time. Many attempts at crisis intervention fail because an adequate historical basis has not been obtained early. It should bring to the surface the salient features of the patient's life, relationships with others, the presenting symptoms, and the precipitants that may have contributed to the crisis state. Organic pathology must be ruled out by history and, if necessary, with appropriate examination and tests. Brain tumors, hypertension, endocrinological disorders, chronic infections, and other organic illnesses commonly present as psychiatric crisis conditions.

Crisis intervention requires greater activity on the part of therapists than do other kinds of psychotherapeutic intervention. Again, because of the tight time frame, the focus on current problems, and the aim of rapid resolution, therapists cannot afford to sit back and wait. Rather, they must be very active from the beginning. Crisis intervenors use suggestion, support, confrontation, and interpretation, as well as organic therapies. They often make interpretations earlier in the treatment process than is the case with other forms of psychotherapy. Hence, crisis intervenors must be experienced therapists who have a full range of psychotherapeutic skills available to them. Experience in recognizing pathology, resistances, and likely etiological factors is necessary.

Crisis intervenors should plan for the termination of therapy from the very onset of treatment. Some time limit or visit limitation should be identified during the very first session. This frequently helps to activate patients who otherwise would dawdle for weeks, months, or even years. A self-imposed limitation on the length of treatment also helps therapists who may dawdle.

Crisis intervention moves through a series of predictable steps. First, the state of panic is stabilized using a combination of medication and support. Second, all available resources are mobilized. Third, the problem is defined while an adequate historical base is established. Fourth, a strategy for solving the problem is mapped out jointly by patient, family, and therapist. Fifth, the planned strategy is implemented.

CONCLUSIONS

There is a good deal of evidence that supports crisis intervention work. Bill[16] looked at different regions in the state of Delaware and showed that regions served by crisis intervention centers had lower hospitalization rates those without such centers. Other studies have yielded similar findings.[17, 18] Greer[19] has shown that crisis intervention discourages suicidal threats and behavior. Straker[20] and Kaufman[21] have shown symptom remission in patients treated with crisis intervention. Langsley, in what is the best controlled study available, showed that social adaptation in crisis intervention cases was at least as good a method as hospitalization.[14]

It is reasonable to suggest that crises present an opportunity for personal growth or personal catastrophe. What happens to people in crisis depends largely on the nature of coping skills, support, and assistance available. Many individuals deal with stress in an acceptable way without assistance or intervention. Others require assistance from families and friends. Still others turn to family physicians or to professional crisis intervenors for assistance with their difficulties. The family physician can develop the skills to assist with crises directly. At the very least, the physician must be able to recognize a crisis and be aware of appropriate referral agencies.

REFERENCES

1. Smith LL: A general model of crisis intervention. Clin Soc W J 4:162, 1976
2. Caplan G: *Principles of Preventive Psychiatry*. New York: Basic Books, 1964

3. Rapoport L: The state of crisis: Some theoretical considerations. Soc Serv Rev 36:211, 1962

4. Bloom B: Definitional aspects of the crisis concept. J Con Psych 27:498, 1963

5. Parad H, Caplan G: A framework for studying families in crisis. Soc Work 5:3, 1960

6. Caplan G: op. cit.

7. Holmes T, Rahe R: The social readjustment rating scale. J Psychosom Res 11:213–18, 1967

8. Paykel E: "Life Stress and Psychiatric Disorder: Applications of the Clinical Approach." In: Dohrenwend BS, Dohrenwend BP: *Stressful Life Events.* New York: Wiley, 1974.

9. Myers J, Lindenthal J, Pepper M: Life events and psychiatric impairment. J Nerv Ment Dis 152:149, 1971

10. Brown G, Birley J: Crisis and life changes and the onset of schizophrenia. J Health Soc Behav 9:203, 1968

11. Mueller D, Edwards D, Yarvis R: Stressful life events and psychiatric symptomatology: Change or undersirability. J Health Soc Behav 18:307, 1977

12. Mueller D, Edwards D, Yarvis R: Stressful life events and community mental health center patients. J Nerv Men Dis 166:16, 1978

13. Sachs VK: Crisis intervention. Public Welfare 26:112, 1968

14. Langsley D, Kaplan D: *The Treatment of Families in Crisis.* New York: Grune and Stratton, 1968

15. Parad H, Resnik H, Parad L eds: *Emergency and Disaster Management.* Bowie, Maryland: The Charles Press, 1976

16. Bill A: The effectiveness of a psychiatric emergency service. Del Med J 41:241, 1969

17. Decker B, Stubblebine J: Crisis intervention and prevention of psychiatric disability: A follow-up study. Am J Psychiatry 129:725, 1972

18. Auerbach SM, Kilmann PR: Crisis intervention: A review of outcome research. Psych Bul, 84:1189, 1977

19. Greer S, Bagley C: Effect of psychiatric intervention in attempted suicide: A controlled study. Br Med J, 1:310, 1971

20. Straker M: Brief psychotherapy in an outpatient clinic: Evolution and evaluation. Am J Psych, 124:1219, 1968

21. Kaufman E, Klagsbrun S: An emergency room changes. Dis Ner Sys, 33:231, 1972

CHAPTER 16

TIME-LIMITED PSYCHOTHERAPY

D. DANIEL HUNT

Counseling or psychotherapy in the family physician's office has long been recognized as a natural part of the physician's interaction. When we define psychotherapy as any interpersonal interaction designed to effect change in an individual's behavior, we at once see the process as encompassing all aspects of the interaction between the patient and the physician. The very manner in which the patient is registered, dealt with during the physical examination, and advised during the prescription of treatment can be seen as a part of the therapy experience. In addition to these aspects of promoting health, there is a place in the primary care physician's office for face-to-face, short-term individual psychotherapy. Balint[1] estimates that fully one-fourth to one-third of the primary care physician's casework consists of psychotherapy. Further substantiating this estimate, a recent epidemiologic survey by Regier[2] reports that 15 percent of the population suffer from some form of mental illness during a 1-year period. Of that group, 60 percent seek and receive treatment in the primary care medical setting.

The goals of therapy in the family physician's office frequently differ from the goals of the mental health specialist. While the psychiatrist may be defining his success by the ability to assist the patient through a reconstructive experience, the primary care physician's goals will be to reestablish the premorbid level of adjustment or modify certain symptoms and attitudes.

Before exploring healing factors within the psychotherapy interchange, it is worthwhile to review the fact that not every physician will be suited to take on short-term psychotherapy cases. The individual who has a need to exert authority, appear omniscient, or who is overly verbose is not suited for the role; he or she is best advised to refer patients to others. It is wise for each potential and active therapist to introspect and to review those traits which promote a healthy engagement and interchange.

CURATIVE FACTORS IN PSYCHOTHERAPY

Several variables contributing to positive outcomes have been identified within the last two decades of research in psychotherapy. While the answers are incomplete there are common characteristics of a relationship which seem to promote healing. The physician who is aware of these various components can maximize their effect.

1. The power of being understood. The therapist requires the patient to organize a presentation; this very process of verbalizing the information frequently sheds new perspectives for the patient. Then, as the patient senses that previously experienced, overwhelming problems can be understood, problems may no longer be seen as unique or sinful. The physician can promote this aspect of therapy by commenting in an accepting and understanding manner.

2. Relationship factors. The ideal model of the supportive therapist can be described as the benign/competent model. Truax and Rogers[3, 4] have suggested that acceptance and accurate empathy, warm positive regard, and genuineness by the therapist contribute highly to positive outcomes. This requires the physician to be real to the patient, and not use the patient for personal satisfaction.

There should be no breach of the professional relationship. In the course of the treatment experience the patient may develop what appears to be amorous feelings for the physician. Frequently, meaningful and careful exploration of feelings reveal them to be related to general attitudes towards authority figures in the past, wishes to truly have and incorporate the help-giving figure, or grateful attempts to repay the therapist's kindness. Other times, these feelings may be attempts to test the therapist's humanity; to see if the therapist really cares. These feelings, as with any other strongly charged emotions, should be talked about and understood in the context of the benign/competent model.

3.   Modeling factors. The therapist conveys a mode of dealing with highly charged feelings which may be new to the patient. Without having to act upon them, the patient's conceptualization of strong feelings and verbalization of them is encouraged. The physician role models this style of dealing with highly charged emotional material.

4.   The factors of "belief in the process." From the work of Jerome Frank[5] it appears that one of the ingredients involved in the healing process is the belief of both patient and therapist that the experience can be of some help. This factor is common to healing relationships formed in cultures very dissimilar to ours. It can certainly be seen in the physician-patient relationship within our culture, and is most clearly demonstrated by placebo treatments.

5.   Educational factors. The educational aspects of the healing relationship range from sharing information to providing a healthy role model. Types of information most helpful are those which take certain behaviors and feelings out of the category of "crazy" or "bad." Obviously, this reeducation is appropriate only after the physician has explored the issue thoroughly with the individual, and is personally reassured that a particular behavior is not an indication of a more serious pathology (for example, recognition with the bereaved that anger may be a part of the mourning process).

Sexuality is another area in which a sensitive exploration and sharing of educational information can be helpful. In spite of real gains in our culture's flexibility for open discussion of sexual development, many individuals live with stereotypic myths about their own and their partner's sexuality. An adolescent with concerns about his sexual identity may be quite relieved to know that masturbation is a normal and healthy sexual outlet. Or, after participating in a homosexual activity, learning that fully one-third of adolescent males participate in some type of homosexual activity (usually group masturbation), can dissipate guilt and fears of homosexuality. Sexual myths are legion and continue into adulthood— the married man fearing masturbation is a sign of marital failure, or spouses who see themselves as sexual failures because of their inability to achieve simultaneous orgasm.

Needless to say, reassurances can only be effective when they follow a careful understanding of the problem. Merely informing the patient of the facts without enlisting confidence and trust will frequently, and paradoxically, discourage further communication and leave the patient with a sense of, "that may be so for others, but the doctor doesn't understand me." More subtle forms of education take place as the patient learns to understand and internalize the nonjudgmental role of the therapist.

6.   Emotional catharsis factors. At work in all helping situations are

the effects of verbal unburdening and consequential emotional catharsis.[6] Catharsis is the outpouring of feelings which have previously been held back. Frequently, people maintain "old tapes" which are so upsetting that they are scarcely acknowledged, let alone verbalized. It is helpful to let these "tapes" receive an airing.

TREATMENT PROCESS

Freud has likened psychotherapy to a chess game. There are a limited number of ways to begin and end. However, the middle process is filled with so many variables and potential moves that no game can be specifically mapped out in advance. It is possible only to specify general guidelines that can then be applied in the family physician's setting.

The section following this one presents guidelines on whom to treat, but first it is important to consider how to treat. The first steps in developing a treatment program are the recognition of problem areas, classification of the difficulties, and finally, the establishment of a treatment contract. Beitman[7] labels this phase the "engagement stage" of therapy. As he outlines, much of the work in this stage revolves around the question, "Can this doctor help me?" Cadoret[8] points out that the engagement interview may be initiated by the physician or the patient as follows:

1. The physician may come across emotionally charged material in the personal history or routine exam which calls for further discussion. If possible, time should be set aside at that point, or an appointment arranged to explore those issues at a later time.
2. Another frequent reason for initiating a longer interview is to explore somatic complaints with no clear organic cause. Questions such as, "Is there something about that symptom that is especially worrisome?" may turn the minor cough into a discourse about a relative dying of lung cancer. Explorations of a recurrent backache may lead to worries about pressures at home, or fears of not being able to hold up at work.
3. The patient may initiate the longer interview with a direct request to discuss an issue with the physician, or with a request for a referral. Any request for a referral to a mental health specialist should be seen as a request for the physician's time and opinion with regard to the problem. The physician can then decide whether to refer the individual or engage directly in a short-term psychotherapy contract.

Following the recognition of problem areas and initial engagement, the second phase takes place, and a prolonged history-taking interview is conducted. Beitman describes this as the "detailed enquiry" period. This involves more than mere history taking. It is the time to search for patterns—recurrent themes in life, persisting from childhood and seen weaving through current symptom-producing experiences. Here the family physician sees the patient in an unhurried period of time (30–50 minutes being most widely used) to better understand the problems and begin an outline of a treatment contract. The number of sessions set aside for this task will vary from patient to patient, and from therapist to therapist. However, it is advised not to use more than three sessions for this phase, and preclude the error of "drifting" into a therapeutic experience without the establishment of goals, time limits, and options.

When families are brought in, longer sessions may be needed; otherwise it is wise to keep within the prearranged lengths of time determined in the initial prolonged history-taking interview. Holding to the agreed upon number of minutes per session conveys the message that there is a specific work space and a specific job to be done. The decisions of how many sessions and what type of fees to levy are also arranged at the conclusion of the prolonged history-taking interview. A short-term contract will usually involve six-to-ten sessions over a 2–3 month period; the understanding is that at the end of that time an assessment of progress will be made and the options for referral, termination, or continuation will be discussed. A useful question to ask in the initial phase is, "How will you know when you are done?" Answers from the patient, like "Getting along better," or "Feeling better about myself," might be acceptable in a long-term approach; but the physician conducting time limited psychotherapy should push the patient to outline more focused and realistic short-term goals. The depressed individual may set the goal of improved sleeping patterns, the anxious person may set the goal of discontinuing the use of minor tranquilizers as a means of coping with day-to-day stress. A phobic individual may focus on being able to cross a specific bridge, or reach a certain height in a building. The explorative exercise of specific goals is useful as it underlines that therapy is both time-limited and problem-oriented. This emphasizes that the patient must actively participate.

The stage of treatment following the identification of patterns and establishment of goals is called "working through." This involves the patient and therapist working together to modify those behaviors or attitudes resulting in diminished patient potential. Working through may involve psychotropic drug intervention, family or couple involvement, or traditional individual therapy.

During this stage, the physician should be aware of the patients' potential to react to the therapist as they have reacted to authority figures in the past. This can be a powerful therapeutic tool; certain patterns can be experienced within the treatment setting. If not recognized, the patients' reactions to authority figures can present a resistance to change, thereby frustrating both parties. These feelings, termed transference, may not develop in the context of the short-term contract. However, it is the sign of an experienced therapist who, when confronted with a confusing and seemingly blocked situation in this stage, considers transference issues.

Short-term therapy is best described as supportive. The descriptive title may imply that it is easy work. This is far from true! It requires a delicate balance of empathic listening in order to quickly engage the working alliance so necessary for any therapy process; at the same time it requires the physician to adopt an active and real role in order to create change in a limited period of time. The work is primarily shoring up defenses and focusing on conscious conflict. Insight or interpretive work is not emphasized unless it clearly mobilizes and assists defensive strengths. The therapist is a real individual in the sense of setting limits and being actively present with constructive feedback.

The role of suggestion and direct advice should be clear in this context. As Balint[1] points out, it is the most often used form of treatment; the real question is not how much is required but how best to utilize it. The most important principle in the use of advice and suggestion must be to caution the physician never to advise or reassure the patient before the underlying problem is clearly identified. Premature suggestion or reassurance may be occasionally successful, but it is more likely to cut off valuable communication leaving the patient with the sense of a real misunderstanding on the part of the physician. The following is an example where a correct but premature suggestion could have closed off communication.

Mr. and Mrs. J. H.

Mr. and Mrs. J. H. had completed an exhaustive infertility workup and learned that Mr. J. H. was sterile. This was discovered late in the workup, as the physician had first proceeded with the wife's workup. Following discovery of the husband's problem, the couple decided to proceed with artificial insemination. Four months into the artificial insemination course the wife presented to her family physician with complaints of backache and abdominal pain. During the examination she revealed that for the first time she was experiencing erratic menses and temperature fluctuations not enabling the period of ovulation to be determined. A prolonged interview touched on a carefully guarded resentment about having to undergo artificial insemination. At this point, reassurance and advice to the patient that she talk to her husband about her disappointment would have probably ended in a dead-end communication. A therapy contract was initiated and in the ensuing 6 weeks it became evident that she feared that her husband would leave her. This was partially due to her anxiety that since he would not be the natural father, he would be less invested in the child should she become pregnant. Once this was carefully explored, she saw more clearly that this was probably not the case. She suggested that her husband join the final session, and they jointly explored their previously unexpressed and mutual disappointments.

In summarizing how to treat, it is clear that genuine empathy and sincere interest in the patient are essential. These qualities, however, are not sufficient for assisting individuals in changing behaviors. What is also required is strategic intervention.

WHOM TO TREAT

The question of whom to treat in the family physician's office and whom to refer to mental health professionals is crucial in determining one's success rate. Incautious selection may lead to a demoralization on the part of the physician and, to use behavioral terminology, extinguish the help-providing behavior. Over and above the following guidelines, the physician's training, interests, and available resources are important variables in the decision-making process of whom to treat and whom to refer. The factor of available time was purposely deleted from this list to emphasize and challenge the physician to review cases in which vague somatic symptoms leading to time-consuming appointments might have been better treated with time-limited psychotherapy.

The discussion of whom to treat brings up the problem of diagnosis. The standard medical diagnostic system often precludes an understanding of behavior and its relationship to symptoms. McWhinney[9]* offers two classifying systems that are used as an addition to the standard pathologically oriented diagnostic model. It is useful to review this diagnostic system to explore who should be treated in the primary care physician's office. McWhinney proposes a taxonomy of patient behavior based on a reference to the doctor-patient contact and one based on contributing social factors. First, the physician establishes a standard medical diagnosis and then considers the questions: "Why is the patient contacting me at this time?" and "What are the social variables involved?" There are five categories for the patient-contact section and seven categories covering social factors. The patient-doctor contact categories consist of the following:

* Reprinted by permission from The New England Journal of Medicine, 287:384, 1972.

1. Limit of tolerance. The patient presents to the physician because his symptoms are causing pain or discomfort that have become intolerable. This covers many straightforward illness episodes such as fractures or colds. Intolerable unhappiness or depression is included here as a symptom complex.

2. Limit of anxiety. The patient presents with symptoms not because they are necessarily intolerable, but because the implications of the symptoms produce an unbearable level of anxiety. McWhinney gives the example of the individual who presents because for the first time he felt his xiphisternum, and comes to the physician complaining of a lump. This is not an example of an inappropriate visit as it reflects the culture's emphasis that lumps should be brought to the attention of the doctor. If, however, the patient fails to respond to reassurance and keeps presenting with different yet similar symptoms, it then can indicate an underlying problem with living.

TABLE 16-1.   Taxonomy of Social Factors in Illness and Patient Behavior*

---

1. LOSS: (a) Personal loss—loss of a loved one through death or desertion. (b) Loss of things—imposed loss of home, cherished possession, job, loss of health or body part.
2. CONFLICT: (a) Interpersonal—conflict within family, with neighbors or at work, where hostility is recognized. (b) Intrapersonal—role conflict or conflicting demands on the patient (as in a working mother).
3. CHANGE: (a) Development—where time of life is the major problem (as in adolescence, menopause or senescence). (b) Geographic—where a move to an unfamiliar environment is the major problem (as in immigration).
4. MALADJUSTMENT: (a) Interpersonal—problems between people with no overt conflict (as in failure to achieve a satisfactory sexual relation without hostility between partners). (b) Personal—failure to adjust to the environment (home or job) in the absence of the above mentioned loss, conflict or change.
5. STRESS: (a) Acute—unexpected event not covered under loss, conflict, or change (for example, the sudden illness of a family member or friend). (b) Chronic—long-term situation not included in loss, conflict, or change (for instance, the presence of a handicapped child in the family).
6. ISOLATION: Not due to any recent loss, change, or conflict (as in an elderly widow).
7. FAILURE OR FRUSTRATED EXPECTATIONS: When the patient's goals in life are not fulfilled; and when there is no evidence of an intervening event covered by loss, conflict, or change (e.g., failure at school or failure to achieve occupational promotion).

---

* Source: McWhinney IR: Beyond diagnosis: integration of behavioral science and clinical medicine. N Eng J Med 287:384–397, 1972.

3. Problems of living presented as symptoms (heterothetic). Episodes of illness that on the surface appear to be straightforward but reflect some problem with the patient's relationship or environment are categorized under this heading.
4. Attendance for administrative reasons. This category covers doctor-patient contacts whose sole purpose is administrative. Here, although the patient is ill, the reason he or she presents to the physician is not for health care but for a certification of the level of disease for third party reimbursement.
5. No illness. This patient-doctor contact covers preventive care visits such as rotuine physical exams or well-baby visits.

The second classification system outlined in Table 16-1 covers the social factors which may contribute to the illness experience. These may be cause, effect, or not related at all, and they focus on the kind of life environment that the individual is presently experiencing. Again, the purpose of adding these two classification schemes to standard medical diagnoses is to sharpen one's eye for potential psychotherapeutic agendas, and to define the groups who might be amenable to counseling. A few examples of the proposed taxonomy will illustrate the use of this system.

1. A middle-aged farmer comes with repeated minor injuries that keep him from working for an unusually long time. It transpires that he hates farming and would like to find other work. Classification—Clinical: Recurrent minor trauma. Behavioral: Problems of living presented as symptoms (heterothetic). Social: Maladjustment (occupational).
2. A middle-aged widow complains of a recurrent dizziness that is not true vertigo. She has just had to admit her mother-in-law, who lived with her, to a nursing home for permanent care. Every time she visits her, she is terrified that the mother-in-law will ask to be taken home. She is given counseling and support, and reports that she is much improved a few days later. Classification—Clinical: Dizziness without organic cause. Behavioral: Heterothetic. Social: Acute stress.
3. A young man with marital problems complains of a small spot on his scrotum. He has recently had extramarital intercourse and is worried about venereal disease. Classification—Clinical: Genital furuncle. Behavioral: Limit of anxiety. Social: Sexual maladjustment.
4. A 28-year-old married woman, known to suffer from multiple sclerosis, attends with blurring of vision. Blurring has been present since her previous relapse 12 months before and has not changed. On further inquiry, it appears that her reason for coming is fear of another pregnancy because her husband refuses to accept birth control. Classification—Clinical: Multiple sclerosis. Behavioral: Heterothetic. Social: Marital maladjustment.

The choice of which individuals to select for time-limited psychotherapy comes from an understanding of the phrase normative crisis. Use of this phrase should in no way lead one to underestimate the serious symptoms which may result from these "passages," "ages," or "developmental phases." The amount of stress and the patient's ability to cope with the specific crisis will determine the level of symptoms. The individuals most suited for a time-limited psychotherapy contract are those whose premorbid level of functioning and interpersonal relationships are relatively good, and whose symptoms are specifically related to the transition from a developmental phase. The goal of the work with this type of patient is to assist in assessing the life position and preparing to move forward. The following case histories illustrate this orientation.

Puberty and Adolescence

B.F. is a 16-year-old high school junior with whom the physician was indirectly familiar through contacts with his mother for weight control counseling. A panicked call from the mother set up the initial family interview. The mother called fearing actual violence in the house between father and son over the recent discovery of the youth's use of marijuana. Over the phone, the family was advised to immediately cease all discussion about the issue until the arranged appointment. The prolonged history taking interview was divided into three segments. First with the family unit, then with the youth alone, and a final discussion with only the parents. From the first segment of the interview, it was clear that all discussion was blocked by each member taking a defensive and rigid posture. The parents were angry and adamant; the young man sullen and totally silent. Enough rapport was established in the boy's private interview to ascertain that the issue had to do with his wish for acceptance in his peer group. His fear was more that his parents' attitudes towards his friends would make him unacceptable to the group. This was demonstrated by their reluctance to have the group over to their house. During this initial exam the young man's tremendous difficulty verbalizing his needs and wishes became evident. The interview with the parents, both of whom were verbal and articulate, gathered the information that B.F. had done average but acceptable work in school, seemed to be slow in forming relationships with his peers, but otherwise had not shown evidence of acting out behavior in the past. The parents confided their fears that B. F., the youngest of three sons, was beginning to resemble their middle son who beginning at 9 had a long history of truancy, theft, and heavy drug abuse. Despite no previous evidence of that level of sociopathy, they rationalized their stern stance by attempting to "cut off at the bud" anything that might develop. The physician, after gathering the data and assessing the case, initiated the six-session contract to formulate a negotiating relationship within the family. In working with this family, it was important to remember the major developmental issues of puberty and adolescence, a period in which the adolescent goes through an apparent chaotic and confusing period because of biologic growth patterns. The identity established in childhood must now be re-hammered and molded with the added pressure of sexual needs. The process involved is for the youth to integrate these forces into a trusted identity conforming to social roles. This identification involves establish-ing a place in the family which is no longer child and yet not quite adult. At the same time, the establishment of relationships with peers is a very important part of this maturational process as the youth begins to naturally grow away from the family.

The therapist used the six sessions to establish communication and support the youth's attempt to articulate his position. This support was often done in a nonverbal manner by moving the therapist's chair next to the young man as he attempted to articulate his needs. At one time this maneuver was used to support the mother. The dictum that all negotiation was to be done in the office was maintained until it was clear that the family unit had a beginning basis to listen to one another. The "contract" negotiated was that marijuana would not be used by the son in return for the parents' guaranty of privacy for the young man. B. F. was given permission to re-do a previously unused basement "rec-room" to entertain his friends. In the end, this project involving the removal of a long unused ping-pong table, putting up Dayglo posters, etc., captured the father's interest and imagination. He was then given B. F.'s permis-sion to join in the renovation project. Over the next 2 years, two more negotiating sessions were established. The first was called by the parents when car use became a mild (though nowhere near as dramatic) crisis, and another called for by the son, when the parents wanted to renege on an agreed upon contract. This last negotiation period was gratifying to the therapist in that he could see that the young man was willing to hear his parents' side, argue his own case, and no longer retreat to sullen detachment.

Young Adulthood

M.S. was a 21-year-old man who was referred back to the primary care physician after extensive neurologic evaluation. This evaluation had fol-lowed the onset of tremor and an abnormal EEG; the patient had a family history of unidentified familial degenerative brain disease. M.S.'s older sister had died at the age of 20 following a 3-year, rapid, and relentless progressive deterioration. The report from the neurologist in M.S.'s case was hopeful in that there was no seizure disorder, and there was a later onset of the tremors than had been the case for the sister. However, little was known about the disorder and M.S. had fallen into a deep depression. He announced his decision to withdraw from the community college in which he was enrolled and a plan to quit his sum-mer job at a restaurant. His mother's understandable concern and tendency towards guilt provided an overprotective environment promot-ing further detachment from outside interests. The prolonged history taking interview revealed significant vegetative symptoms of depression consisting of early morning awakening, a diurnal variation, diminished appetite, weight loss, and significant anhedonia. A concern about his own sexual identity was touched on during this interview, as was his loss of peer group support after his inability to continue with tennis. An 8-week contract was established and antidepressants begun. The normative quality of his reaction was supported by the therapist.

In this phase of life, the youth has hopefully established a sense of self, and must now work on intimacy and avoid isolation. Intimacy, in this case, should be seen both as a capacity to form partnerships and commitments to concrete affiliations. The primary care physician is reminded that the majority of individuals pass through all of these phases without need for assistance, but those who experience added insult may be vulnerable to such pitfalls as detachment and isolation at each phase of maturity. It is at these points of crisis that short-term counseling can be most effective.

For two of the sessions, the physician and patient left the office to walk on a wooded path to discuss the various issues haunting this young man. This latter gesture proved to be very helpful in allowing M.S. to establish a trusting working relationship. The contract was renegotiated after 2 months to include medication follow up and longer sessions at monthly intervals. While the total answer is not in yet, and M.S. continues to live with the possibility of deterioration, he has resumed his college coursework and depressive symptoms have abated.

Adulthood

Mr. B.T. can be best described as a man "lost in time." At 46 he was still driving a cab for a large company, having never settled into one of apparently many potential careers. His own anxiety-forestalling defense of seeing himself as tremendously capable but just never discovered, was reinforced by his taxi patrons' enthusiasm for his well-informed opinions and plans for executive career roles. Unfortunately, the stories of his plans to have impact on the system were only updated to fit the current political or economic situation—action never followed. Gradually, as years passed and potential doors closed, a chronic depression settled in. In understanding this patient it is important to keep in perspective the development issues of adulthood. Erikson[10] describes the central theme during this maturational period as the struggle for generativity versus stagnation. This is the concern in establishing and guiding the next generation, as well as creating a productive and satisfying role within the cultural norms that provide the basic necessities. Hopefully, by this point in a person's life he has established an ability to form intimate relationships. Typical problems during this phase have to do with child rearing, career directions, and goals as predominant and recognizable themes.

Back pain first brought Mr. B. T. to the attention of the physician. Given the lack of vegetative symptomatology, antidepressants were not indicated, and an eight-session counseling course was embarked on. Here, the therapist used the first two sessions to engage Mr. B. T. by listening carefully to his futuristically oriented plans. In the third session the therapist continued in a reality-oriented mode, but he confronted Mr. B.T. with his years of waiting. This was an attempt to get the patient to deal with current problems. The depression worsened. A mid-week call from his wife concerned with his sense of hopelessness and suicidal thoughts prompted an earlier than scheduled appointment. This was a potential turning point. The first third of the session was filled with the patient's sense of failure as the myth of his ability to eventually become a "great man" was breaking down. The therapist's role was a crucial one of providing a sense of support and helping the patient to deal with his feelings of alienation. At the same time, the therapist was careful to avoid over reassuring the patient and colluding in the rebuild-ing of a myth which had for so many years staved off real change. The remainder of that session was used to help the patient explore his assets and remaining potentials. Clearly, his premorbid loquaciousness and entertaining manner served him well in his years driving the cab. Over the course of the following five sessions a decision was made by Mr. B.T. to purchase his cab and begin as an independent operator. Follow-up appointments at 6 months and 1 year saw him winking to the therapist about his "great plans for the future," but he was clearly on his way to a more realistic goal; his fleet of cabs had grown from one to three in that 1-year period.

Maturity

Mrs. E.S., 72, initiated contact with the physician for counseling. The prolonged history taking interview outlined many lonely experiences and an increasing fear of dying alone. The interview revealed that Mrs. E.S. was long widowed and had three grown children. There were no vegetative symptoms of depression. The perplexing part of the puzzle was the distance this lady traveled. Each visit entailed a 4-hour round trip. While flattered at her insistence that the particular therapist was the only one who could help, the physician was reluctant in agreeing to a six session, monthly contract. The reluctance stemmed, in part, from a lack of specific goals for the outcome. An attitude of "let's try it and see" was adopted with the developmental issues being kept in mind. Erikson describes possible outcomes of this last phase of maturation as "ego integrity or despair."[10] The successful outcome of this transition is the organization of the past into a personally meaningful experience tak-ing into account accomplishments, failures, people, and possessions. This personal organization must provide a means of dealing with death. The approach of death in this phase is not intangible, or a philosophical ex-perience as it was in earlier periods and adulthood. It is now a real and palpable presence as the individual experiences day-to-day pain, failing organs and grief over other significant losses. The ability to pursue this while maintaining self-respect is the goal. The individual who is unable to cope with this and fails to integrate these issues experiences despair.

After Mrs. E. S.'s third visit, the improvement was striking and the physician's curiosity was piqued. Mrs. E.S., with considerable embar-rassment and great tact explained that while she enjoyed the 40-minute discussions with the doctor, her real joy came in anticipating the regular trip to the appointment. This involved her oldest, unmarried daughter who lived in the same town as her mother and who picked her up and drove her to the city in which the "therapy" took place. The mother and daughter then stayed overnight with the youngest daughter and the grandchildren in the same city. A brief telephone discussion with the daughters found they also enjoyed this contact. The monthly visits were therefore formalized during a family meeting. Future monthly visits wisely excluded the physician.

The final stage in therapy is termination. Terminating work with a patient is at times as difficult for the therapist as it is for the patient. The patient's feelings about the termination should be noted and brought up for discussion several sessions before the planned end. These feelings can be useful in the ongoing process, as they reflect how the individual deals with other losses. For those individuals for whom the time-limited approach has not been enough, the groundwork for a referral would have been laid in the initial session; and hopefully it will not come as a blow to the patient's sense of self-esteem.

Often a goal of time-limited therapy is set to help an individual assess what he or she wants to work on in preparation for referral to a mental-health specialist. This can serve to bridge the transfer of care in an effective and empathic way, thereby assuring the involvement of the patient with the new therapist. Other patients involved in time-limited therapy will find relief, reach goals, or gain tools to carry on alone or by infrequently visiting the physician/therapist.

The termination stage may be a period in which previously resolved symptoms briefly flare up. It may be helpful to point this out in advance. Instances of separation during the treatment process, such as the therapist's vacation, may reflect and predict issues within the termination stage.

Appointments for three-month or six-month followup can be a mutually beneficial experience. For the patient, it provides a way to touch base with the physician; the feedback to the physician assures his or her own growth and maturity as an effective therapist.

CONCLUSIONS

Facets of the physician's personality have been linked by psychotherapy research to positive outcomes. These variables of genuineness, accurate empathy, and sincere interest encourage the engagement and provide the base on which change can be made. Strategies recommended are time-limited in nature with one to three sessions for establishment of realistic goals, and six to twelve sessions to work toward that end.

The choice of patients is important; individuals with a good premorbid level of functioning who currently experience symptoms secondary to normal developmental transitions are the most amenable to this approach. Formulation of goals with the developmental milestones in mind helps the therapist and patient contract for focused and obtainable goals. Involvement of appropriate family members or the patient's spouse in a working contract is encouraged when appropriate. It is equally important to establish an end point so that progress, or the lack of it, may be assessed and strategy changes made.

REFERENCES

1. Balint M: *The Doctor, His Patient and the Illness.* New York: International Universities Press, Inc. 1972
2. Regier DA, Goldberg ID, Taube CA: The de facto U.S. mental health services system. Arch Gen Psychiatry 35:685, 1978
3. Truax CB: Effective ingredients in psychotherapy: An approach to unraveling the patient-therapist interaction. J Counsel Psychol 10:256, 1963
4. Rogers CR: *Client Centered Therapy.* Boston: Houghton Mifflin, 1951
5. Frank JD: *Persuasion and Healing.* Baltimore: Johns Hopkins University Press, 1973
6. Wolberg LR: *Short Term Psychotherapy.* New York: Grune & Stratton, Inc., 1965
7. Beitman B: Engagement techniques for individual psychotherapy. Soc Casework 60:306–309, 1979
8. Cadoret RJ, King LJ: *Psychiatry in Primary Care.* St. Louis: C. V. Mosby Co., 1974
9. McWhinney IR: Beyond diagnosis: Integration of behavioral science and clinical medicine. N Eng J Med 287:384, 1972
10. Erikson EH: *Childhood and Society.* New York: W. W. Norton and Co., Inc., 1963

CHAPTER 17

FAMILY THERAPY

DONALD C. RANSOM AND NICHOLAS T. GRACE

This chapter presents concepts and methods that are central to the field of family therapy. It begins with a selective look at the historical context of family therapy. Next, the field is defined and its purposes are outlined. Reasons to use or not to use this approach are next discussed. Some principles and techniques are spelled out to introduce the language of family therapy and then a case illustration is presented.

HISTORICAL BACKGROUND

The history of family therapy runs a parallel and occasionally interconnected course with the changing emphasis on the role of the family in health, illness, and care. From the field of social work, Zilpha D. Smith said the following in 1890: "Most of you deal with poor persons or defective persons as *individuals*, removed from family relationships. We deal with the *family* as a whole, usually working to keep it together, but sometimes helping to break it up into units and to place them in your care."[1]

At the first round-table discussion of the American Orthopsychiatric

Association in 1930, Charlotte Towle added to her predecessors when she remarked that "Treatment cannot be given to any member of the family without affecting the entire group. In some cases, the entire family must be drawn into treatment. Approach to this or that member or centering treatment on a certain individual cannot be a random thing."[2] The prolonged discussion that followed at the round-table focused largely on whether notes should be made in front of the patient. No reference was made to Towle's earlier remarks and her formulation was left unexplored. Family relationships were left on the periphery of mental health concerns, where they remained for the next 20 years.

The modern history of family-centered health care begins with "The Peckham Experiment."[3-5] What began in 1926 in South London as a "family club" with some health screening benefits had grown by 1935 into the "Pioneer Health Centre," housed in a three-story, 58,000 square-foot structure. "It was a great venture: a social structure to be built with a new unit—not the individual, but the family."[5]

From the beginning, the aim was to construct a setting "designed to be furnished with people and their actions."[5] It was a biologist's living laboratory, not a medical clinic; an experiment the purpose of which was to study life *in vivo* and thereby study health rather than illness. For this purpose it was well equipped, housing a large swimming pool, gymnasium, game rooms, a music room, library and quiet room, work rooms, nursery, a large dance floor with stage, a theatre, a self-service cafeteria and pub, a store, and outdoor grounds, eventually expanding to incorporate a summer camp and a cooperative farm 7 miles away. Enrollment reached 1,400 families, all living within a mile ("walking distance") in the principally lower-middle class and middle-class neighborhood. The War brought an end to the Centre in 1939.

Two features of The Peckham Experiment stand out in the context of this chapter. First, the project had a well-developed conception of the family.

> Before beginning to build, it is necessary to know what bricks are to be used, or in modern terms, what must be the *unit* of construction . . . We claim to have defined the unit of Living. It is not the individual; it is *the family*.[5]

The second feature of The Peckham Experiment is that deliberate structures were devised for seeing whole families together in consultation. The primary mechanism was built around the "Family Health Overhaul" and the "Family Consultation." These involved doing a history and physical examination for each individual, including basic laboratory analysis and exploration of family health and social life. The unique feature, which has not been matched in sophistication to this day, is that the re-sults were shared with the group, with an eye toward constructing ave-nues for change from the outset.

As The Peckham Experiment drew to a close, "The Study of the Family in Sickness and Health Care," supported by the Josiah Macy, Jr. Foundation, was just beginning. This study was a cooperative venture among members of the faculties of Public Health, Medicine, and Psychiatry at Cornell University Medical College, and representatives from New York Hospital. A group of fifteen families was studied over a 2-year period with the goals of: (1) understanding "the interrelation between illness and the family situation;" (2) learning something about the "implications for treatment" that followed from such an approach; and (3) "exploring the best methods for cooperative treatment" with the family health care team assembled for the study. The report of that study, *Patients Have Families*, was prepared by the project's director, Henry B. Richardson, and published in 1945 by The Commonwealth Fund.[6]

The Macy Study was aware of The Peckham Experiment and drew upon it. What the British group provided in commitment to the family as "the unit of living," their American counterpart matched with a conceptually powerful description of the family and its processes. Supported by detailed case analyses, *Patients Have Families* presents the unmistakable notion of the family as a system operating to regulate the health and illness of its members. The first two parts of the book, "The Family as the Unit of Illness" and "The Family as a Unit of Treatment," attest to the clear grasp of the family as a biosocial unit. An appendix presents such concepts as "focus," "polarization," "reciprocating systems," and "factions," which are forerunners of many family system processes regularly described and studied today.

It is ironic that the family system approach was formally proposed for the general medical audience before it made its great breakthrough in psychiatry and mental health. The presentation in *Patients Have Families* anticipated the psychiatrist Don Jackson's famous (1957)[7] notion of "family homeostasis" by 15 years. The Macy team did not realize the full implication of their conceptual advance for clinical work; they remained hampered by traditional habits. It was the team, meeting together periodically, that tried to put the family picture together, building a composite of different perspectives and points of contact. They did not stress the importance of bringing together the whole family for purposes of either gathering information or working directly on interpersonal relations. This was to be the great breakthrough to come from practicing psychotherapists. Modern medical care has traveled a long route to find its way back to the important contribution of The Macy Study and The Peckham Experiment.

From mid-century to the present, family therapy has grown rapidly and spread out in many directions. The field is now so large that its different pathways cannot be adequately summarized here. Synoptic histories of developments within the past 25 years can be found in Block and LaPerriere (1973),[8] Bowen (1975),[9] and Guerin (1976).[10]

DEFINITIONS

Family therapy is both a form of therapeutic intervention and a conceptual approach to psychopathology and behavioral problems. As a form of therapeutic intervention, family therapy is not a treatment method in the usual sense. There is no agreed-upon set of procedures followed by practitioners considering themselves family therapists, and no set of techniques to which they strictly adhere. Different therapists approach different families in a variety of ways.

As a conceptual approach to psychological, behavioral, and medical problems, family therapy embodies the family approach. In its simplest statement this means that problems are understood and addressed primarily as aspects or expressions of social relational contexts, rather than as properties of individuals, abstracted from their recurring patterns of ordinary daily behavior.

A definition of family therapy that combines focus and purpose is as follows: *Family therapy is the process of working at the level of human behavior bounded by intimate relationships, with persons having a history and a future together, in order to influence an agreed-upon problem.* This definition purposefully stretches the everyday meaning of the word family to a special type of relationship, instead of a particular entity. There is no question that marriage and the family are formal institutions, different from and usually more important than other forms of human association. Yet, people are also involved in other intimate relationships, holding membership in groups that rival the family in intensity, duration, satisfaction of needs, and impact on health. Family therapists work with people who hold a wide range of ties with one another; a workable definition of family therapy should reflect this scope.

The proposed definition also uses the terms influence and problem instead of cure and illness. Family therapy has very little connection with the mental illness model; the purpose of therapy is to introduce changes that take place between people, rather than administering treatments for an individual's disease. Expanding on this emphasis, family therapy is concerned with four types of problems:

1. Individual problems in which other family members are viewed as contexts involved with the expression of one member's symptoms, such as illnesses, pain, anxiety, behavioral abnormalities, and misbehavior.
2. Problems between pairs of persons, such as parent-child, siblings, or marital tensions, in which both the larger family and its more limited aspects are viewed as context.
3. Family problems per se in which the group is unable to achieve its shared goals, is unable to supply its members' basic needs, or misuses its members.
4. Problems between one part of the family and another, or between the family and representatives of the community such as the school, medical providers, or the legal system.

To properly qualify this outline of the problem types, it is useful to draw a distinction between two vantage points: the therapist who for practical reasons can decide what a problem is and who has it; or the therapist who can decide what a problem is for purposes of establishing some higher truth in the matter. The question is, who is to say what the "real" problem is when a patient presents with a symptom, and how can it ultimately be known who is "really" involved? To say that an individual is the problem is arbitrary, but may be useful for purposes of proceeding with therapy. To say that the marital pair or the family is the problem, and that an individual's behavior is only a symptom may also be useful, in another instance. The important observation is that the act of defining a problem one way or another is a point of therapeutic leverage, not philosophic truth-seeking, and it depends upon a combination of the therapist's style with the unique circumstances of every case. It is therefore a political act in the grandest sense of the term, not a revelation of fact brought about through medical or psychological discovery.

INDICATIONS AND CONTRAINDICATIONS

Because family therapy is both a conceptual approach and a form of therapeutic intervention, it is not to be viewed as simply another treatment tool indicated for some problems, but not others. One always "thinks family" (Sluzki, 1974),[11] and any kind of therapy is a way of intervening into a family. Whether one works with an individual or with multiple members of a family, from the family therapy point of view the reality of mutual interdependence still remains. The remaining question is whether one works directly with the family in an implicit or explicit manner.

One reason not to work directly with the family is strategic. For example, a therapist can be attempting to influence family relationships by working directly with only one member of the family. Although the group is the unit of intervention, the individual who comes to the office becomes the primary agent of change in the therapeutic process. This approach usually involves seeing all relevant members of the family together at least once before deciding to work intensively with any one member.

Other reasons for not working directly with the family are all in the category of impractical or unworkable. In sum, the family approach is always indicated. How that view gets operationalized into practical work is limited only by the therapist's imagination.

Common Presentations in Office Practice

An important question is whether there are indeed particular conditions that respond more successfully to family therapy than to other forms of intervention. Unfortunately, there is little systematic research; and data are not available to answer the question. However, it has been suggested on the basis of clinical impressions, that family or marital work is the response of choice for several problems or clinical presentations. The following list presents the most important of these:

1. Marital and sexual adjustment problems which are presented as such in the office.
2. Family problems brought up in the office as needing attention: intense sibling rivalry, intergenerational conflicts, or serious disagreements about child-rearing.
3. Any problem involving children that is greater than a self-limiting or common illness; adjustment reactions of childhood.
4. Serious problems of teenagers involving separation and the achievement of independence.
5. A crisis or chaos in the family that is not being well handled and may lead to further distress or symptomatic behavior.
6. When one person claims the problem is caused by another, for example excessive drinking or being house-bound.
7. When any member of the family shows signs of mental or emotional disturbance.
8. When any member develops a stress-related illness.
9. When intervention requires life-style changes affecting or involving members of the family, for example a radical change in someone's diet or daily life rhythm.
10. When a serious, chronic illness or disability in a member is not being handled well by the family.

11. When medical symptoms are present for which no organic basis can be found.
12. When other forms of treatment have failed.

PRINCIPLES AND TECHNIQUES

Following is a brief description of thirteen key concepts, techniques, and terms central to family therapy. Some language and tools will be introduced to prepare the reader for the case discussion to follow.

Individual versus Family Focus During the Conjoint Sessions

Some therapists focus on the inner world of past learning, wishes, motives, coping strategies, internalized representations of the world, and the like. Others focus on the outer world, the demands it makes, and the contradictions and problems it poses. Therapists seem to have a natural preference, a kind of empathy or identification with one side or the other. Family therapists are divided on this issue. The authors' view is that both worlds are needed to understand any person, family, or problem; the two sides make up an essential equation. We are only beginning to understand the relationship between inner and outer.

The Family as a System

Perhaps the single most important concept in family therapy is that of the "family-as-a-system." Today, terms such as homeostasis, morphostasis, and self-regulation through feedback are used to describe the family's dynamic properties. A key idea centers around the importance of wholeness; the notion that the family is an emergent whole that can never be known from the knowledge of only the individuals who compose it. A second key idea is mutual interdependence, in the sense that all members of a system are linked together in mutual influence; a change in one member of the system must be accommodated (adapted to) by other members. The root metaphors involved are those of context and ecology. Nothing can be understood or changed except in relation to everything else with which it is in essential association.

The "Identified Patient"

The idea of the family as a system is abstract, and the danger of its application is reification. In the early days of family therapy, a kind of axiom developed which stated that the real problem is the family, and

The net result was that the seat of pathology was shifted from the indi-
the individual only behaves symptomatically as the "identified patient."
vidual to the group. The motivation for this conversion was positive, but
therapy was often begun by attempting to persuade the group to adopt
the new view. The problem with this tactic was that it required the
therapist to induct those involved into a particular belief system as a pre-
condition of therapy. It is now widely accepted that special inductions
are not needed to begin successful therapy. Rather, two levels of thinking
are kept distinct—at one level the therapists's theoretical convictions, and
at the other level the definition of the situation that is actually shared
with the family in order to proceed. It is suggested, therefore, that the
widely known concept of the identified patient be used cautiously and
selectively, if not totally abandoned.

Diagnosis

Diagnosis in family therapy bears little resemblance to diagnosis in traditional psychiatry, but shares much in common with the diagnostic process of modern family practice. Little emphasis is given to categorization;
great emphasis is placed on identifying and describing significant problems. When formal diagnosis is done, it is usually for institutional or insurance purposes; most third-party payers will only reimburse expenses
for "treatment" of individual patients with diagnosed "mental illness."
The failure to recognize families as legitimate units of health care, and to
acknowledge that intimate relationships can be the source of human mal-
functioning is an anachronism that at last shows signs of changing.

A central idea in family therapy is that diagnosis is not the identification of what the patient has, like measles; it is the construction of a
definition of reality that can either help or hinder the process of change.
Thus, the labeling of a problem or a family process is itself a strategic act.

History

Family therapy focuses on the present situation and recurring patterns
of behavior between persons. The past is not explored unless the present
cannot be understood, or unless the therapist thinks the family can best
discuss the present if it is framed in the past.

Group Focus

In family therapy, the focus is directed to issues of common concern
and/or to problems existing between the members present. Ideally, the
therapist initiates a sample interaction between or among those present.

For example, it is useful to ask those present to discuss a problem, come to a decision, or plan something together. A more elaborate example is the "family sculpture" sequence described in the case that follows. The data derived from directly observing interpersonal behavior is significantly different from data derived from listening to self-report.

Flexibility about Whom to Include

Although the theoretical framework favors dealing with whole families, the decision about whom to include in formal sessions is handled flexibly by most therapists. It depends upon who is available to bring together, and what the therapist wishes to accomplish. Close friends, a clergyman, or a probation officer might be included. Even family pets have a place in therapy at times. Some therapists like to see larger groups and do what is called network therapy. A minimum of thirty persons might be set for the meeting to proceed.[12, 13] Other therapists see groups of four or five families together and call it multiple family therapy.[14]

Minimal Therapy

Family therapy as illustrated here exercises the principle of minimal therapy. The principle holds that it is the therapist's job to make the least possible intervention needed to allow the family's own health-enhancing capacities to work freely again. Therapy may be brief or long-term, depending upon the circumstances. Ideal times to intervene are in moments of family crisis when the therapist can help the family avoid mishandling a difficult situation. However, this principle is tricky for it is sometimes not clear whether resolving a crisis or reducing a symptom has solved the problem, or perhaps only restored the family to a previous level or type of functioning (homeostasis). This once again sets the stage for a repetition of the sequence that reactivates the symptom or crisis just resolved (recursiveness). One must simply wait, watch, and be available to move quickly and more knowledgeably if there is a reoccurance. The physician in family practice has the advantage of a continuing relationship with a likely knowledge of meaningful change.

Problem Focus

The principle of minimal therapy applies well when the therapist sees his role as one who joins with a family to clarify and solve problems. In the process of solving problems, organizational changes, insights, and meaningful emotional experiences may occur that allow the family members to grow; but these are side effects from the primary work of resolving problems.

In contrast to this approach, there is a substantial portion of the family therapy field that defines its goals differently. Instead of the solution of specific problems, there is an emphasis on personal growth and the expansion of life's potential. The growth approach is educational, interpretive, and experiential. It proceeds as if what people really need is something other than, or more than, relief from the complaints they came in with. For example, it focuses on explorations of how people feel about one another, or suggests exercises to develop awareness and communications skills.

Giving "Homework"

Family therapy is an action-oriented therapy whose work is divided between what happens in the formally arranged sessions with the therapist, and what is directed to go on in the time between. Thus, therapy goes on around the clock, and between sessions through the medium of directed assignments. Giving tasks to individuals and families has several purposes:

1. Directives are designed to introduce change into habitual patterns of behavior, thereby leading to different subjective experiences.
2. Directives provide behavioral samples to be reviewed in the formal sessions. These samples are current, and the therapist has a hand in organizing them. The less productive alternative is to talk about the past or about something with which the therapist has no direct involvement.
3. By assigning tasks, the therapist becomes involved in action outside as well as inside the formal sessions. The relationships with those involved are thereby intensified, and kept very much alive in the time between sessions.
4. Giving homework is a way of gathering information. Each assignment is like a diagnostic probe. How people respond to requests designed to lead to desired changes provides invaluable information. It instructs the therapist as to what issues are important and how to proceed with the next step.

Designing and giving homework embodies a basic premise: it is the therapist's responsibility to formulate the strategy of change that patients wish to achieve, and to carry out that strategy through assigning tasks. The therapist initiates an action, and anticipates what might happen. Through feedback the therapist then learns what actually happened, which in turn leads to the design of the next step to be taken. In this mode, responsibility for change is not totally on the patient. The therapist is not passive and often initiates patient activity.[15]

Alliances and the Coalitionary Process

A coalition is an agreement of alliance established for the mutual benefit of the allies vis-a-vis a third party. It is arrived at by explicit negotiation and/or by implicit cues provided by the context and by the interaction itself.[16] For some therapists, working with the coalitionary processes between members of a family and between individual family members provides the core of family treatment.

This universal process in social life has been described in a variety of terms, including family triangles.[17] In the case presented later a central issue was the triangle between mother, son, and father. A primary goal of therapy was the alteration of the observed triangle by means of an alliance established by one of the therapists and the mother. It is common strategy in family therapy to establish shifting, instrumental coalitions for purposes of facilitating change, while managing not to get locked into binding coalitions.

Reframing

To reframe, according to Watzlawick, Weakland, and Fisch, "means to change the conceptual and/or emotional setting or viewpoint in relation to which a situation is experienced and to place it in another frame which fits the 'facts' of the same concrete situation equally well or even better, and thereby changes its entire meaning."[18] Reframing offers the possibility of introducing a change while the situation itself may remain quite unchanged and indeed, unchangeable. What is changed as a result of successful reframing is not the concrete facts, but the meaning attributed to the situation, and therefore its consequences. Thus, the meaning of an adolescent's behavior can be reframed from that of a disobedient, thoughtless, budding juvenile delinquent to that of a young man seeking greater personal autonomy. The process is word magic, but it must respect the laws of plausibility and good faith if it is to succeed.

Visibility

The family sessions described later were observed by a number of residents and teaching staff who also participated in discussions of what went on and what was to happen next. There is always the danger of having too many cooks in the kitchen, but we wish to emphasize the openness and visibility of family therapy to all concerned members of the family as well as professional colleagues who can help or learn from the experience.

AN ILLUSTRATIVE CASE

There is tremendous variety in family and marital therapy, and disagreement from within the field on the best ways to proceed. These differences are best revealed through observation of styles and technical procedures actually utilized in practice. The case presentation that follows stands on its own as an example of the authors' style of family therapy. It also serves to illustrate certain principles and techniques described in the previous section. This particular example is chosen because the therapy took place in a model family practice unit, and because the case involves both a behavioral and a medical problem in two different family members; thus demonstrating how intervention at the family level can simultaneously resolve both types of problems.

A 16-year-old boy, the oldest of four children, was referred by his school counselor to a family psychiatrist. During the preceding 6 months the boy had been cutting classes, misbehaving in school, and swearing at a teacher. This infuriated his father, whose efforts to get him to "shape up" not only failed, but were followed by an ever-worsening situation. The boy's behavior at home had also become a problem. The son and his father had become so alienated from one another that the father was threatening to place him in a foster home. It was upon this note that the counselor recommended family therapy.

Dr. B saw the family for the first time in his office; the second visit was scheduled for the Family Practice Center. Four weekly sessions were held there, and a brief follow-up session was held 1 month later. The following account is a summary of what was discovered, the problems that were addressed, the major techniques that were used, and how intervention proceeded.

The first session was devoted to gathering information and formulating problems that could serve as the target for therapeutic intervention. All six members of the household were present: mother and father, in their late 30s; their 16-year-old son; two daughters, 12 and 10; and a 2-year-old son. Quite naturally, the father focused on the misbehavior of his son. The mother agreed that their son had been acting terribly, but she seemed more sympathetic than the father. As she talked, she seemed to say that she was stuck in the middle between her husband and her son; yet she did not come right out and put it in those words.

Mrs. A was obviously suffering from the strain of recent events and about 20 minutes into the session Dr. C, who had joined Dr. B as co-therapist, decided to make an alliance with the mother and work toward bringing her some relief. Mrs. A agreed to do a "family sculpture" with the assistance of Dr. C (see Duhl, Kantor, and Duhl, 1973, for a primer in the sculpting method employed here).[19] He took her to the middle of the room and explained that her task was to arrange the members of her family around her in whatever locations and postures she chose: a representation in living sculpture of how her family felt most of the time to her. Mrs. A's creation was instructive. She essentially portrayed her stuck-in-the-middle and frustrating position in the family.

After observing the pose, Dr. C rearranged the group's seating pattern. He pulled Mrs. A out and invited her to join him across the room, suggesting that it might prove helpful to everyone to have her out of the middle of things for a while. As the group talked, it became clear that as relations between father and son deteriorated, they talked more and more through Mrs. A and less directly to each other. Further exploration revealed that Mrs. A had suffered with ulcerative colitis for a long time. The problem was flaring up again. A visit to the gastroenterologist earlier in the week had involved discussing the possibility once again of a surgical procedure.

As the hour drew to a close, family homework for the next session was assigned. The first directive was designed to detriangulate mother, son, and father. Mother was instructed not to be an intermediary for any information passed between the son and father, nor to be a sympathetic listener for either one's complaints. Father and son were to deal directly with each other. In addition, Mrs. A was to be relieved of all disciplinary obligations toward the son, and was told only to do those things with him which were mutually enjoyable.

A negotiation process between father and son was then initiated to build some supportive structure around their renewed contact. The most important thing the father wanted from his son was for him to go back to school without cutting classes or swearing at teachers; in short, just to put up with school for a while, even if he didn't like it. In exchange the son asked for complete freedom of movement with the stipulation that he would tell his parents where he was going, whom he would be with, and when he would be back. The father agreed and the session ended on this note.

A week later everyone met again. Mrs. A looked better. She said she had easily lived up to her part of the bargain. It also turned out that the son and father had entered into competition over who could outdo the other in living up to their agreement. The boy had not missed any school and had also made up a week's work. He had not been late once in coming home at an announced time. He had done all his household chores without a single reminder, and had even done the dishes twice for his sister. Mr. A was being studiously respectful of his son's new freedom, and had volunteered to pick him up and drive him home from any place at any time. The session lasted half an hour and was spent reviewing the homework and answering questions about it. No further explorations were made, and no explanations of why things seemed to be working were undertaken. The directive for the next session was to continue the previous assignment with one addition. At some time during the week, J and his father were to do something together, that both would enjoy. Exactly what that would be was up to them. We asked to see only Mr. and Mrs. A the following week.

One week later, Dr. B began the session by saying that as families grow, there is a natural expansion of the father-mother role that can crowd out the husband and wife role. He further explained that it is sometimes useful to separate various components of the family from the whole, especially the marriage partners. This permits a focus on the parent as a couple; confirms the reality of their relationship within the larger, overshadowing family life process. The introduction set the stage for the discussion that followed. First the past week was reviewed. Everyone had continued to carry on the new pattern and it was beginning to feel like the norm rather than an experiment. Father and son had spent Saturday together, and while it was enjoyable, Mr. A reacted strongly that it was not right to spend time with just one member of the family. The family always engaged in recreation as a group; Mr. and Mrs. A had not even been out together for an evening alone for seven and a half years.

When asked when he felt his very best, Mr. A replied, "On Sunday morning when the whole family is seated together in our pew at church." He explained that although he was not a religious man, the whole family's presence symbolized something very important to him. Sunday mornings had become a point of contention in the family. For some time now, J had refused to go to church at all. Mrs. A went reluctantly about half the time; she dreaded going and felt miserable while she was there. For Mrs. A being in church together symbolized the opposite of its meaning for her husband. She said that some of her happiest moments were when the rest of the family was in church and she was home alone for a couple of hours, sitting around in her bathrobe doing nothing, but enjoying the peace and quiet.

It was clear that Mr. and Mrs. A had been in conflict for years over "family togetherness," and had not resolved the issue. That was not pointed out or commented upon. There was no need; the family awareness was far keener than the therapists'.

The session closed with a directive. Mr. and Mrs. A were to go out to dinner alone sometime during the next week. During that time they were to think of each other as husband and wife rather than as mother and father.

One week later, the whole family met for the last regular session. J was going to school, doing well, and living up to his word on every occasion. Mr. A decided that J should get his license and drive the family car. J was hardly mentioned again. The discussion turned to Mr. and Mrs. A and their evening out. It had been a bit awkward, but enjoyable. Mrs. A looked like a different person from the one first seen 3 weeks ago. She said that she did not know what to make of it, but two and a half weeks ago her bleeding episodes had stopped and her gut pain had let up and not returned. She had not felt better physically in years.

Most of the hour was spent talking with Mr. A. He had many questions—about family closeness, fatherhood, and how other families strike a balance between being together and being separate as individuals. It was as if he could imagine for the first time that members of his family were also individuals, and that there might be other ways to be a family than the one he had always struggled for. But he did not know what these alternatives were or how to go about trying them out. At this point, the purpose of some of the events of the past few months was reframed. It was suggested that all families go through a process of working out what it means to be a loyal and proper member of one's family, and what it means to be a person in one's own right in relation to the rest of the world. 16-year-olds in particular are constructing a sense of their own independence and separateness from the family, and this always leads to conflict and pain. In the A family, not only was J working out his own individuality, he was working for the family, especially his mother. J was trying to push back the limits of what was acceptable and break down some long-standing rules of family conduct. Part of that work involved "blowing the whistle" in some fashion so that some agency outside the family was drawn in or forced to get involved. Otherwise the family was stuck, unable to change itself. Everyone was cautioned that this was just one way of looking at what had been happening, not the gospel truth, or what "really" happened. The interpretive framework was to be taken with a grain of salt.

A brief meeting one month later and a follow-up call one year later confirmed that all was well, including Mrs. A's problem with chronic ulcerative colitis.

CONCLUSIONS

Family therapy is both a conceptual approach to a wide range of problems and a body of techniques designed to influence relationships. Its point of therapeutic leverage is changing what happens between people who have great meaning to each other. The strategy of family therapy fits well with the family practice model. With appropriate training, all family physicians should be capable of conducting formal family therapy sessions with a wide range of patients.

While all family physicians benefit from a family approach to comprehensive health care delivery, the decision to offer formal marital and family therapy services is up to each individual. The kind of work described in this chapter makes special demands on the provider, personally and practically, in relation to running a practice.

For those readers desiring to do family therapy in office practice, some closing words of encouragement and advice are offered. First, develop a good family charting system. Family problems and interactions are of a different logical order than individual problems and personal behavior; a good record system is capable of recording both levels of reality (see Grace et al., 1977,[20] and Medalie, 1978,[21] for examples). Second, choose a regular time slot in the weekly schedule when all members of the families to be seen can come. This usually means an evening or a Saturday morning. Finally, no matter how much one may wish to do family or any other type of psychotherapy, there is always more to do than time allows. Referrals will be necessary. In addition to time constraints, referral is the best choice when there is a conflict of interest, such as when the patients involved are personal friends and the provider might be manipulated into choosing sides. Another instance for referral is when the problem presented is beyond the scope of what the primary provider thinks he or she can handle. Cultivating a good working relationship with at least one therapist who can be counted on is highly recommended. In time, that relationship will prove to be an invaluable outside resource.

REFERENCES

1. Rich M: *Belief in People.* New York: Family Service Association of America, 1956
2. Towle C: "Treatment of Behavior and Personality Problems in Children: The 1930 Symposium, The Social Worker." In: *Orthopsychiatry 1923–48.* New York: American Orthopsychiatry Association, 1948
3. Pearse I, Williamson GS: *The Case for Action.* London: Faber & Faber, 1931
4. Williamson GS, Pearse I: *Biologists in Search of Material.* London: Faber & Faber, 1938
5. Pearse I, Crocker L: *The Peckham Experiment: A Study in the Living Structure of Society.* London: Allen & Unwin, 1943
6. Richardson HB: *Patients Have Families.* New York: Commonwealth Fund, 1945
7. Jackson D: The question of family homeostasis. Psychiatr Q supplement 31 (part 1), pp. 79–90, 1957
8. Bloch DA, LaPerriere K: "Techniques of Family Therapy: A Conceptual Frame." In: Bloch DA, ed: *Techniques of Family Psychotherapy: A Primer.* New York: Grune & Stratton, pp. 1–20, 1973
9. Bowen M: "Family Therapy After Twenty Years." In Dyrud J, Freedman D, eds: *American Handbook of Psychiatry.* New York: Basic Books, Vol. 5, 1975
10. Guerin PJ: "Family Therapy: The First Twenty-five Years." In Guerin PJ, ed: *Family Therapy: Theory and Practice.* New York: Gardner Press, 1976
11. Sluzki C: On training to "think interactionally." Soc Sci Med 8 (9/10) 483–485, 1974
12. Speck R, Attneave C: *Family Networks.* New York: Pantheon, 1973
13. Rueveni U: *Networking Families in Crisis.* New York: Human Sciences Press, 1979
14. Laquer HP: "Multiple Family Therapy: Questions and Answers." In Bloch DA, ed: *Techniques of Family Psychotherapy: A Primer.* New York: Grune & Stratton, 1973

15. Haley J: *Problem-Solving Therapy.* San Francisco: Jossey-Bass, 1976
16. Sluzki C: The coalitionary process in initiating family therapy. *Family Process,* 14:67–78, 1975
17. Bowen M: Family psychotherapy. Am J Orthopsychiatry, 31:40–60, 1972
18. Watzlawick P, Weakland J, Fisch R: *Change: Principles of Problem Formation and Problem Resolution.* New York: W. W. Norton, 1974
19. Duhl FJ, Kantor D, Duhl BS: "Learning, Space, and Action in Family Therapy: A Primer for Sculpture." In Bloch DA, ed: *Techniques of Family Psychotherapy: A Primer.* New York: Grune & Stratton, 1973
20. Grace NT, Neal EM, Wellock CE, Pyle DD: The family-oriented medical record. J Fam Pract 4:91–102, 1977
21. Medalie J: "Family History, Data Base, Family Tree, and Family Diagnosis." In Medalie J, ed: *Family Medicine: Principles and Applications.* Baltimore: Williams & Wilkins, 1978

SUGGESTED READING

The following eight books are recommended for anyone wishing to pursue further how to think about and how to do marital and family therapy.

Bloch DA, ed: *Techniques of Family Psychotherapy: A Primer.* New York: Grune & Stratton, 1973
Guerin PJ, ed: *Family Therapy: Theory and Practice.* New York: Gardner Press, 1976
Haley J: *Problem-Solving Therapy.* San Francisco: Jossey-Bass, 1976
Laing RD: *The Politics of the Family and Other Essays.* New York: Pantheon, 1969
Minuchin S: *Families and Family Therapy.* Cambridge: Harvard University Press, 1974
Napier AY, Whitaker CA: *The Family Crucible.* New York: Harper & Row, 1979
Paolino TJ, McCrady BS, eds: *Marriage and Marital Therapy: Psychoanalytic, Behavioral and Systems Theory Perspectives.* New York: Brunner/Mazel, 1978
Papp P, ed: *Family Therapy: Full Length Case Studies.* New York: Gardner Press, 1977

CHAPTER 18

USE OF FAMILY HEALTH GROUPS

ELLEN McGRATH AND RAYMOND C. ANDERSON

ROLE OF GROUPS IN FAMILY MEDICINE

Family physicians should be natural group counselors. Theoretically and practically, no other specialty in modern medicine has the opportunity to deal with group phenomena as frequently as family medicine. Diagnoses in family medicine consider not only the pathophysiology of illness, but also the role of the patient's family, social environment and feelings, and their effect on health problems. Attention to people's health in relationship to primary groups (i.e., the family), highlights the need for family physicians to develop a working knowledge of group and sociological phenomena.

Recognition of these needs has led to the recent development of behavioral science curricula and experiential training as a typical part of family practice education. This increased emphasis on studying psychological and social processes raises important questions of (1) What modalities are appropriate to the armamentarium of the family physician? and (2) Is competence as a counselor a legitimate goal in the training of family physicians?

On a theoretical level, the importance of group concepts is generally recognized in the teaching of family medicine. For example, in a typical family medicine text, *Family Medicine: Principles and Applications,*[1] the entire first section of the book focuses on the impact of different levels of group phenomena in family practice. This section deals with group themes such as identifying family and community characteristics, and how social patterns and sociological processes impact on a family's health.

There is also a successful historical precedent and context for using groups in direct patient care. In 1907, Pratt,[2] a general physician, began using group experiences in his work with tuberculous patients—he achieved such success that the psychiatrists in mental hospitals were stimulated to try group techniques in the 1920s. Not only were group approaches used with patients, but they were used as a learning device for physicians. Freud[3] used a group to develop and conceptualize psychoanalysis with his Wednesday Evening Society meetings. The theory of psychoanalysis nurtured and matured as this group met for over 2 years.

Despite the importance of group phenomena and sociological principles in family medicine, most family physicians continue to use a one-to-one model of patient care. This lack of group implementation tends to occur because family physicians have experienced little, if any, specific training in group theory and process. Many family physicians also feel uncomfortable with the traditional psychiatric context of group work.

Family physicians actually have more group experience than they may first realize. The experience of physicians in their own families, their work in hospitals, in medical schools, and in community events can provide valuable knowledge about groups. For example, family physicians are significantly more "nurtured, affiliative, and introspective" than physicians in other specialties.[4, 5] These are the very qualities associated with effective group leadership styles.[6]

Recently, a trend has emerged where physicians are applying group techniques to patients with similar physical problems. These new groups deal with a wide range of health problems typically encountered in family medicine. A variety of psychophysiological problems treated in groups has been described by Blake,[7] Pomerleau,[8] Wollersheim,[9] and Abramson.[10] Group assertion techniques for alcoholics have been used with significant success.[11, 12] Groups have also been utilized quite effectively with the terminally ill, such as those dying of cancer[13] and with the mothers of leukemic children.[14] A wide range of physically handicapped children and adults have been treated in groups, even toddlers who have delayed speech and language development.[15] With the belief that group support enhances rehabilitation more than other approaches, San Francisco Veteran Administration personnel have used group approaches extensively in the rehabilitation of vascular surgery patients. Groups help the amputees with their feelings of helplessness, isolation, and depression; and make the staff more aware of the particular management issues for these patients.[16]

Group process has also been applied to normal developmental issues. Deutsch and Kramer[17] used groups to help the elderly understand that aging is a normal part of the life cycle. The development of more positive attitudes helped the elderly help themselves. In keeping with the current change in childbirth procedures, groups are used to teach Lamaze methods and to counsel pregnant couples. Once the child has been born, groups have also been used more frequently for couples to develop effective parenting techniques. Men who accompany women seeking legal abortions[18] have been placed in clinic groups for counseling at the same time the individual women are receiving abortions, and Burnell[19] has described groups for women after the abortion has occurred.

In an attempt to systematize group approaches in family medicine, Friedman, Jelly, and Jelly have recently written four sequential articles[20-23] in which an experienced therapist works with the family physician as a co-leader for the group. However, the authors do not distinguish between group psychotherapy, which takes a number of years to learn and a certain amount of supervised clinical experience, and the kind of group approaches which family physicians could readily use without adding greatly to their current experiences.

This distinction is an important one; the family physician's training in psychotherapy is usually quite limited. Group psychotherapy works to identify and change emotions and, sometimes, personality styles of patients. The approach requires a knowledge of psychopathology and specific clinical experience in conducting psychotherapy. While group psychotherapy as described by Friedman et al.[20-23] can be learned by family physicians, their co-therapy model may be time-consuming. It may involve psychiatric knowledge and skills which most family physicians do not feel are of great practical use.

Other group approaches do exist, however, whereby several principles of group psychotherapy and group process can be applied readily, practically, and effectively by family physicians. The family medicine groups are not therapy groups per se; they are educational groups in which some therapeutic experiences occur. These groups are particularly well-suited to family physicians since they do not require a great deal of additional reading, clinical experience, or clinical supervision. In addition, these groups utilize the personality characteristics and skills commonly found in family physicians.

To summarize, the therapy groups proposed by Friedman et al.[20-23] provide a more advanced step in the developing technology of family medicine groups. For most family physicians, a simple group model is more readily applicable to a family practice, clinic, or department; this model involves Family Health Groups (FHG's). The FHG's are short-term, educational experiences which explore one topic related to the health needs of patients and their families. They use a group discussion format which encourages patients to share experiences and solve problems. Informational handouts on the specific topic may be used.

Groups typically run from 4–6 weeks, and should have between five and eight members. If the group is started with less than five people, it is less stable and group process can be more complicated to handle. If more than eight people are accepted, the principles of small group dynamics change, and the dynamics of large groups must be applied. If the group stays between five and eight people, a "family" environment is created that can be used by the family physician for enhanced learning in the group. With five to eight people, group members will often assume a variety of family roles with each other, such as mother, father, or siblings, and the group will more closely assimilate real life experiences.

SETTING UP AND CONDUCTING FAMILY HEALTH GROUPS

1. *Establish Goals for the Group.* FHG's can be run by the family physician alone or in a co-therapy model where the family physician works with a colleague or someone from another discipline (e.g., a nurse, physician's assistant, psychologist, or psychiatrist).

Common goals for FHG's include (1) education and understanding of the relationship between physical and emotional experiences in producing health problems for families and individuals; (2) provision of opportunities for interpersonal experiences to resolve health/illness issues and generate support for patients; (3) help patients learn to give and receive feedback and develop more effective communication skills; and (4) encourage patients to assume responsibility for themselves and the quality of their health by teaching self-care methods.

2. *How to Select Members for Family Health Groups.* Several articles have discussed how to select suitable people for group approaches.[18, 20–27] Most of these studies focus on the leader's assessment of the potential group member's use of interpersonal skills for learning. The patient must have at least minimal skills to communicate and listen to others. The patient need not be aware of the cause of his or her problem, even if these problems are interpersonal and/or health-related conflicts. Patients who express interpersonal conflict through psychosomatic symptomatology may be especially well-suited for group work in family practice.

Slavson[25] suggests that the group patient must have a certain amount of "ego strength," that is, the patient must be able to give and receive feedback, and still maintain some sense of self. Horwitz[26] agrees with Slavson, but from a slightly different perspective. He states that "the most general consideration relates to the issue of the patient's capacity to stick with treatment." Horwitz suggests that the patient must be able to tolerate the frustrations of group experience which do not typically occur in the one-to-one doctor-patient relationship. These group frustrations include more instances of delayed gratification, less attention focused on the particular individual, and a greater tendency to lose individuality as each member's identity and needs merge more with the group.

The family physician must also make global assessment of the degree of psychopathology in potential group members. If the patient is unable to function in a primary aspect of his/her life, then the patient should be referred to a mental health professional for psychotherapy. Other contraindications for group therapy include the following:

1. Slavson[25] indicates that people who have experienced intense sibling rivalry, or have very poor control over their feelings and behavior are not appropriate for group.
2. People with psychotic or significant neurotic conflicts are not appropriate for group (this area includes those who are having direct reactions to certain trauma, such as the recent death of a close relative or friend).
3. Patients with transient situational disturbances, such as an immediate crisis, may be more appropriate for crisis intervention or individual counseling.
4. Friedman[27] adds that people who are significantly depressed, especially those with suicidal tendencies or gestures, are clearly not indicated for group.
5. Psychopaths, schizoid, very hysterical or paranoid personalities, and people who heavily monopolize interaction are also inappropriate for group.

Patients particularly well-suited for FHG's are those who share a similar psychosocial-physical problem. Examples include excessive weight loss or gain, alcoholism, other substance abuse problems, chronic diseases such as asthma or diabetes, hypertension, people who have experienced similar physical traumas such as heart attacks or ulcers, or those with similar developmental tasks such as pregnant couples or menopausal women.

To achieve a homogeneous grouping, the family physician must develop a system to identify patients with similar health problems. This can be done by maintaining an index card file system. Each card includes the basic information necessary for a group referral (age, sex, marital status, family members, cultural background, and a brief list of the patient's major physical and psychological problems.) Patient cards are filed according to their major presenting symptoms. Sections could be developed for such problems as alcoholism, weight gain, smoking, heart disease, cystic fibrosis, diabetes, developmental delays in children, gerontology issues, pregnancy, menopause, and headaches. When a topic section is filled with five-to-eight cards of people with similar concerns, the cards can be pulled and people contacted for a group screening interview. This procedure would also facilitate inter- and intra-office and clinic group referrals, so patients could be readily redistributed and referred, depending on group openings with physicians in the same family practice or in nearby clinics.

It is important that the family physician encourage the patient to play an active role in the selection process. Lieberman, Yalom and Miles[28] emphasize the value of patient selection before entering a group, rather than having to make an ultimate decision to drop out. Early dropouts are considered an unequivocal failure in group psychotherapy.[29] Premature termination can reinforce feelings of inadequacy and exacerbate the patient's health problems.

Premature termination also has a detrimental effect on the remaining members of the group. Ideally the group leader hopes to maintain fixed membership in the group (the same members attend each week). Fixed membership is critical in producing more positive group outcome and building group cohesiveness; one of the best tools the family physician has for promoting exploration and resolution of health issues.[30] Fluid membership in groups, with people moving in and out of the group, tends to make everyone more anxious and considerably less productive, since they must constantly focus on changing membership boundaries. The importance of attendance should be discussed with the patients in the initial screening interview.

3. *Conducting the Initial Screening Interview.* The initial screening procedure is very important for diagnostic reasons, as well as to insure that the patients are quite clear about the purpose and structure of the group. Screening interviews must be done on a one-to-one basis with the group leader. In this way, the interviewer can build trust with patients; individual questions and concerns which may get lost in the larger group process can be answered.

A number of issues are faced in the screening interview. Group leaders may find patients resistant to groups; they feel the group has a psychological connotation which does not apply to their particular "physical" health problem. Groups also provide a more anxiety-arousing situation for most people than didactic interactions of a one-to-one nature; the feedback in groups is more diffuse, and the opportunity for judging the effectiveness of the communication is not as clear and available.

There is also an expectation in groups that people will get lost and their needs will not be met because of so many people competing for supposedly limited resources. Old ghosts of sibling rivalry frequently appear as a resistance to entering a group. Another typical resistance involves the feeling that the patient is basically inadequate to be able to support and help others. These group resistances should be watched for in the initial screening interview. If identified, the physician can reassure and inform the patient of the positive and supportive nature of groups.

4. *The Importance of Group Boundaries.* An orientation which encourages patients to take responsibility for themselves in joining a group, requires that the physician provide adequate information about the how, what, why, and where of the group. In short, the family physician must be clear about group "boundaries." Boundaries are defined as anything that limits and/or defines a particular situation or event. Group psychotherapy literature and organizational research has shown that groups cannot be effective unless boundaries are identified and maintained by the leader in a clear, consistent, but not rigid manner.[31]

Examples of important boundary issues include a regular meeting place, the fee, billing and payment procedures, group punctuality, its duration over weeks, group goals, the kind of health focus for the group, expectations of behavior for the leader and for the members, a general sense of the composition of the group, and what to expect of them.

There is also a "content" boundary in groups. This involves keeping the topic of discussion as close as possible to the goals of the group. It is usually helpful to focus on and reinforce feelings, rather than thoughts; encourage people to talk about their own experiences, rather than other people's experiences; keep the discussion in the here and now, rather than on the past histories or people no one else knows; and help the group members to focus on giving and receiving direct feedback to each other.

In summary, boundary issues can and should be discussed at the initial screening interview and at the beginning of a group, so that everyone understands the boundaries and agrees that the group is an experience they wish to have. The initial screening interview should also orient the patient to how groups work[32] and what can be expected in a group.

An article by Gauron and Rawlings,[32] "A Procedure for Orienting New Members to Group Psychotherapy," provides excellent guidelines, and is a useful handout for group orientation. Skills are described for effective problem-solving in groups. They question "I am as I am" statements as ways to avoid change. Historical excuses or reasons for the present problems are fruitless discussion topics. Blaming others for current problems is a way to avoid taking responsibility. The leader should not present advice, or provide solutions to others; they should help members explore all their alternatives, and analyze the consequences of their behavior. The leader wants to talk about behavior that can be seen as specific and relevant. The leader wants to avoid being judgmental, focus on positive as well as negative behaviors.

Gauron and Rawlings also describe eight basic ground rules for group sessions and their boundaries. These can be summarized as follows:

1. Focus on the present, the here and now, and reactions to each other in the group.
2. Be equally committed to helping others as well as yourself.
3. Be honest, talk straight.
4. Discuss feelings as well as thoughts.
5. Listen to all members carefully.
6. Try new behaviors and take responsibility for changing your own behavior.
7. Confidentiality is critical in a group—everyone agrees not to discuss group experience outside the group, unless it is a self-concern.
8. Groups are most effective when all members participate.

5. *Time, Place and Fee Boundaries.* Groups typically run from 1 hour to 1½ hours, depending on the leader's preference. The groups can be run anytime during the day, or during lunch or early evening, if most members work outside the home. Each of the participants should be requested to make a time commitment to attend all sessions (4 to 6 weeks).

Location can be quite flexible, as long as there is space for everyone to sit comfortably. The office waiting room of the family physician may be an ideal setting for these groups,[20] as long as there is no traffic at the time. Interruptions by people entering or leaving, or interruptions by phone must be avoided. In general, group leaders prefer that patients sit unobstructed in a circle or semi-circle. This increases the leader's and members' ability to observe nonverbal responses.

Group fees can range from the regular family practice fee for the amount of time the group will take, to the typical fees charged by group practitioners in a particular community.

6. *Family Health Group Leadership and Membership Boundaries.* It is especially important that role and behavior expectations be explained to potential members. Role expectations for patients include the following:

1. Patients will explore as openly and honestly as possible their feelings and ideas related to the discussion topic for that particular group.
2. Patients will attempt to give and receive feedback about what they observe and feel with each other and with the group leader.
3. Support and shared problem-solving will be encouraged for all members.
4. If readings are used, patients will complete the reading for the next group.

Expectations for the group leader could be:

1. The group leader will model and facilitate communication and learning regarding emotional and physical health issues.
2. The leader will make the group as supportive a place as possible, so the members will feel trusting and open to problem-solving.
3. The leader will be prepared each week with a topic for discussion, and readings or handouts related to that topic.
4. The leader will make an attempt to start on time and focus on the discussion topic, thereby enabling the group to work as efficiently as possible.

7. *Leading a Family Health Group.* The first group session can begin by introductions of the leaders and all the members. Then, each participant can be asked what he or she hopes to gain from the group. Time and place boundaries, member and leader expectations, and group goals can be briefly reviewed to initiate a shared sense of purpose and immediately increase group cohesion. In that way, everyone knows what to expect, there is a shared commitment to the goals of the group, fear of the unknown is lessened, and effective group work can occur more quickly.

In terms of specific styles to adapt as a leader, rely on your own intuition, and your training and experience as a family physician. In one of the better articles on group leadership, Lieberman[6] describes "what leaders do." Leadership conduct includes evocative behavior, coherence-making, support, managing behavior, and use of self. The most effective leaders are those who focus on feelings, and provide support and warmth. Lieberman calls these leaders "the providers" and "the energizers." The least effective leaders are those who are very structured or very unstructured, rigid, and emotionally distant. These leaders are called "the impersonals," "laissez-faire," and "managers." Lieberman summarizes his findings thus: "The most effective leadership style would combine moderate stimulation [from the leader to the group], high caring, use of meaning attribution, and moderate expression of executive function [i.e. establishment and maintenance of boundaries]. Conversely, the less effective leaders are either very low or very high on stimulation, are low on caring, do very little meaning attribution and display too little or too much executive behavior."

One way for the group leader to provide "moderate stimulation" and "meaning attribution" for the group is to differentiate between group content and group process. The group process is the meaning behind what is being said and/or acted out in some nonverbal behavior. When a member talks about a particular topic, the group leader listens with "a third ear," listens not only to what is being said, but also to what it might mean and the context in which this topic is being discussed. Since FHG's are educational groups rather than therapy groups, the leader's task is to use group process mainly to gain a clearer understanding of what the patient feels. The FHG leader does not interpret the patient's behavior or feelings to reveal unconscious motivation, as would occur in group therapy. The therapist is not concerned with why the patient feels a particular way, or how the patient's feelings may be connected to other aspects of subjective psychological experience. Rather, group process is used as an effective tool for the FHG leader to help patients identify what they really feel about health issues; plans can then be formulated for behavioral change, and changes in behavior will eventually cause feelings to change.

An example of attention to group process follows:

A particular group member complains at length about the variety of doctors he has seen; the member is uncertain that his current doctor is "right" for him. Most group members would be likely to respond on a content and advice-giving level. They might make suggestions about how to find a "good" doctor or refer the patient to one of their own doctors. The group leader can take the members a step further. The leader thinks not only in terms of problem-solving, but also in terms of process: what the person really feels about finding a "good" doctor, what was said before this person spoke, and what occurred in the group to which the person may be responding. Also the leader would question if this person's comment reflects a general behavior pattern of complaining behavior and passivity which is dysfunctional for the person.

When the group leader has a clear and persistent idea about the feelings associated with a patient's statements, the leader could say, "It's clear you have had some very disappointing experiences with doctors. How do you express your disappointment and frustration? Was this way of expressing your feelings constructive for you?"

At a deeper level and with more trust between the patient and leader, the leader might suggest, "I wonder if some of what you're saying has to do with a fear you have of some kind of sickness which perhaps no doctor could possibly treat. Sometimes when people have difficulty finding the right kind of doctor, it has to do with a feeling that they are a hopeless case, and even if they could find the right doctor, there's probably nothing that can be done.

The above examples illustrate process rather than content responses by the leader. With experience, a group leader can think more frequently on the two tracks of process and content, and learn to make comments which will further the work of the group by encouraging an expression of true feelings. Identification and acceptance of feelings, in addition to problem-solving or intellectual sharing of thoughts and experience, will make the group significantly more effective.

8.   Evaluating the Group. Group evaluation is an important part of group leadership functions. During the group, the leader can stop the discussion at an appropriate point and ask members to evaluate how "our group is going," and whether members' needs are being met. If not, how can "we" change the group to more appropriately meet our needs. This approach shares responsibility with the patients for the quality of the group; it reminds them that the leader does not have all the power and cannot "save" them.

Evaluation of the entire group experience proves useful for both the leader and the patients. One way to approach this task is to ask patients to list their goals before the first group session. At the end of the sessions, the leader asks the patients to rate how well they accomplished their goals and why. General questions concerning the experience can be written out in the last session and impressions discussed in the group. Questions for the evaluation form can include: What was most helpful in the group? Least helpful? What would you most like to change? Suggestions for future group topics and/or experiences? Strengths and weaknesses of the leaders and of yourself in the group. Another approach is to ask patients after each session to list the most important events for themselves in that particular group and discuss why these events were of importance.

Only through some type of pre- and postgroup evaluation can the leader gain any real perspective concerning the complexities of groups. Evaluations will identify what was useful and gratifying, or what was dysfunctional for both the leader and the patients. The evaluation data can then be used to readjust future groups in terms of structure, leadership style, and topics for discussion. Eventually a practical, efficient, and effective model for FHG's will evolve.

CONCLUSIONS

In summary, recognition of the difficulties in evolving new group models needs to be appreciated. Groups are complex. In many ways, group work is more difficult than one-to-one patient contact. Initiating groups involves significant risk-taking for inexperienced leaders, but eventually, a leader gains enough experience to really appreciate the tremendous rewards inherent in group work. For many types of chronic health problems, as well as practical preventive medicine, groups can be far more challenging and rewarding than the one-to-one contact most physicians experience.

A careful survey of existing evidence indicates that group approaches are significantly effective in patient care.[33–37] Groups have been particularly useful in treating common health problems.[7–11] Despite this evidence, most family physicians remain skeptical as to the utility of groups in their particular practice or clinic. Why bother to set up a referral system, screen patients, and schedule another hour or an hour-and-a-half to see a group? Most physicians are already over-extended in their time commitments, and an FHG seems like an unnecessary, additional burden. The answer to such doubts is efficiency. It is more efficient to see five to eight people with a similar health problem for an hour or an hour-and-a-half, than to see each patient individually. FHG's emphasize health education and preventive medicine, so the number of return visits for patients may be considerably less. Office staff also can be used more efficiently. Registered nurses, physician's assistants, social workers, etc., can be trained to run FHG's. (Despite this efficiency, the authors encourage physicians to run some groups themselves; the effectiveness and personal rewards in working as a group leader are particularly gratifying.)

The challenge of group work can be made considerably easier and more gratifying if the physician works with an experienced group leader as a co-therapist. It may be useful to set up regular or periodic group supervision with a mental health expert in group work. The supervising person can directly observe the group (occasionally or regularly), and then discuss group process possibilities with the physician.

In terms of relevant readings, one of the most useful books for inexperienced leaders is Yalom's *The Theory and Practice of Group Psychotherapy*.[30] Two journals which contain practical and innovative approaches to group therapy are *International Journal of Group Psychotherapy* and *Small Group Behavior*.

Despite available reading and supervision, Family Health Groups are a new idea. The benefits of the approach to physicians and patients would seem to outweigh any costs or disadvantages. The task for physicians is to develop the skills and group structures which particularly fit the needs of family practice.

REFERENCES

1. Medalie JH ed: *Family Medicine: Principles and Applications.* Baltimore: Williams & Wilkins, 1978

2. Pratt JH: The principles of class treatment and their application to various chronic diseases. Hosp Soc Serv 6:401, 1922
3. Freud S: *Group Psychology and the Analysis of the Ego.* London: Hogarth Press, 1953
4. McGrath E, Zimet C: Female and male medical students: Differences in specialty choice selection and personality. J Med Ed 52:293, 1977
5. McGrath E, Zimet C: Similarities and predictors of specialty interest among female medical students. J Am Med Wom Assoc 32:361, 1977
6. Lieberman MA: "Behavior and Impact of Leaders." In Solomon LN, Berzon B, eds: *New Perspectives on Encounter Groups.* San Francisco: Jossey-Bass, 1972, Chap 8
7. Blake A: Group approach to weight control: Behavior modification, nutrition, and health education. Perspect Pract 69:645, 1976
8. Pomerleau O, Bass F, Crown V: Role of behavior modification in preventive medicine. N J Med 292:1277, 1975
9. Wollersheim J: Effectiveness of group therapy based upon learning principles in treatment of overweight women. J Abnorm Psychol 76:464, 1970
10. Abramson E: A review: Behavioral approaches to weight control. Behav Res Ther 11:547, 1973
11. Adinolfi A, McCourt W, Geoghegan S: Group assertiveness training for alcoholics. J Stu Alcohol 37:311, 1976
12. Haberman PW: Factors related to increased sobriety in group psychotherapy with alcoholics. J Clin Psychol 22:229, 1966
13. Yalom ID, Greaves C: Group therapy with the terminally ill. AM J Psychiatry 134:396, 1977
14. Kartha M, Ertel I: Short-term group therapy for mothers of leukemic children. Clin Pediatr (Phila) 15:803, 1976
15. Colman MD, Dougher BA, Tanner M: Group therapy for physically handicapped toddlers with delayed speech and language development. J Am Acad Child Psychiatry 15:395, 1976
16. Lipp MR, Malone ST: Group rehabilitation of vascular surgery patients. Arch Psy Med Rehabil 57:180, 1976
17. Deutsch CB, Kramer N: Outpatient group psychotherapy for the elderly: An alternative to institutionalization. Hosp Community Psychiatry 28:440, 1977
18. Gordon RH, Kilpatrick CA: A program for men who accompany women seeking legal abortions. Community Ment Health J 13:291, 1977
19. Burnell GM, Dworsky WA, Harrington RL: Postabortion group therapy. Am J Psychiatry 129:220, 1972
20. Friedman WH, Jelly E, Jelly P: Group therapy in family medicine: Part 1. J Fam Pract 6:1015, 1978
21. Friedman WH, Jelly E, Jelly P: Part 2: Establishing the group. J Fam Pract 6:1243, 1978
22. Friedman WH, Jelly E, Jelly P: Part 3: Starting the group. J Fam Pract 7:317, 1978
23. Friedman WH, Jelly E, Jelly P: Part 4: A case report. J Fam Pract 7:501, 1978
24. Grunebaum H, Kates W: Whom to refer for group psychotherapy. Am J Psychiatry 134:130, 1977
25. Slavson SR: Criteria for selection and rejection of patients for various types of group psychotherapy. Int J Group Psychother 5:3, 1955

26. Horwitz L: Indications and contraindications for group psychotherapy. Bull Menninger Clin 40:505, 1976,
27. Friedman WH: Referring patients for group psychotherapy: Some guidelines. Hosp Community Psychiatry 27:121, 1976
28. Lieberman MA, Yalom ID, Miles MB: *Encounter Groups: First Facts.* New York: Basic Books, 1972
29. Nash E, Frank J, Glideman L, Imber S, Stone A: Some factors related to patients remaining in group psychotherapy. Int J Group Psychother 7:264, 1957
30. Yalom ID: *The Theory and Practice of Group Psychotherapy,* 2nd ed. New York: Basic Books, 1975
31. Colman AD, Bexton WH, eds: Group Relations Leader. Washington, D.C.: A. K. Rice Institute, 1975
32. Gauron EF, Rawlings EI: A procedure for orienting new members to group psychotherapy. Small Group Behavior 6:293, 1975
33. Pattison EM: Evaluation studies of group psychotherapy. Int J Group Psychotherapy 15:382, 1965
34. Cabral R, Paton A: Evaluation of group therapy; correlations between clients' and observers' assessments. Br J Psychiatry 126:475, 1975
35. Cabral R, et al: Patients' and observers assessments of process and outcome in group therapy: a follow-up study. AM J Psychiatry 132:1052, 1975
36. Corsini RJ, Rosenberg D: Mechanisms of group psychotherapy: Processes and dynamics. J Abnorm Soc Psychol 51:408, 1955
37. Dick BM: A ten-year study of outpatient analytic group therapy. Br J Psychiatry 127:365, 1975

CHAPTER 19

USE OF COMMUNITY RESOURCES

MERRILL N. WERBLUN AND REVA K. TWERSKY

Family physicians accept the responsibility of providing comprehensive health care for their patients. This means care for the physical, emotional, sociological, and rehabilitative needs of patients and their families. To carry out this responsibility, the family physician needs (1) to appreciate the interrelationships between physical disorders, social environment, and psychosocial disorders; and (2) to recognize that it may be necessary to reach out to appropriate resources available in the community. It is this second issue with which the present chapter is concerned.

In any community there exists a composite of health resources which physicians need to identify and integrate into their practices. To successfully accomplish this task, family physicians should be familiar with the roles of other health professionals as well as with roles of various community agencies. Also critical to the effective utilization of community resources is the physician's ability to set realistic expectations when referring patients. Finally, the physician who makes a referral to a community agency wants to remain an active participant in the continuity of care. Thus, the physician functions as facilitator and coordinator of all aspects of the health care system. This is best carried out by (1) making an appropriate assessment of need; (2) facilitating the referral to the appropriate community agency; and (3) evaluating the agencies utilized.

MAKING AN APPROPRIATE ASSESSMENT OF WHAT IS NEEDED

Identification of How the Patient/Family Perceives the Problem

A clear understanding of the patient's presenting complaint, how the problem is perceived by the patient, and previous attempts on the part of the patient or family in utilizing community resources are key to developing an appropriate referral to a community agency. A complete assessment of the problem may require more than one office interaction.[1, 2] It is important that the physician remember to expand an understanding of the patient's problem, to include assessment of what it is the patient is asking for, and what the patient will accept. Failure to identify these areas can lead to an incomplete assessment and utilization of inappropriate community resources.

Case History

Ms. M, an 83-year-old woman depressed, frail, and living alone, complained of increasing difficulty in taking care of her apartment. Rather than exploring this in more depth with the patient, the physician felt that a retirement home or senior citizens housing project would meet the needs of the patient. Arrangements were made for the patient to visit a low-cost retirement home, as well as a senior citizen housing project. The patient did visit these and politely expressed appreciation to the agencies involved. She refused to move to either one of them.

Following the failure of this referral, the physician arranged for a social worker to visit the patient at her home. The home visit revealed the patient's great pride in her long-time residence, filled with family heirlooms. An assessment of need revealed that a neighbor did the grocery shopping for the patient, the apartment manager was available for other needs, and all that the patient really wanted was someone to do heavy cleaning. An appropriate referral was made to a public welfare agency for "chore services." This provided the patient with 2 to 3 hours per week of help and alleviated her major concern. Additionally, through a senior services organization, arrangements were made for an outreach worker to periodically visit the patient for ongoing evaluation and support. These regular contacts also provided the patient's socialization needs.

In this case a proper assessment of need revealed that the patient was asking to remain in her own home, surrounded by personal objects. Her desire was to continue to be as independent as possible. The resources needed to help her achieve this were indeed available, once they were successfully identified.

Identification of Available Support Systems

Identification of the patient's available support systems will often determine the appropriate utilization of a community resource. The physician should turn first to those support systems available within the nuclear family or extended family of the patient. Often through the use of a family conference, the physician can identify strengths and support which are available to the patient. These will determine the appropriate utilization of a community resource.

Case History

Mr. T at age 55 suffered a cerebrovascular accident which left him aphasic and physically incapable of caring for himself. The physician caring for Mr. T in the rehabilitation unit recommended to his wife that he be placed in a nursing home. This suggestion was unacceptable to the patient's wife. The family physician then held a family conference with the wife and children; he carefully identified for them the patient's limitations, physical needs, and prognosis. Attention was paid to the fact that the wife was not capable of managing her husband by herself. During the conference it became clear that the children were concerned and willing to help in their father's care. The physician also found that within the family there existed enough financial support to develop a home care program.

After identifying available support people, the physician specified the care needed, and facilitated the acquisition of appropriate equipment for the home. A social worker facilitated a referral to a home care organization. This organization provided for home health aides who would assist in the care of the patient. The success in answering the needs of this particular patient was based on the physician's ability to identify support people within the nuclear family and appropriate outside agencies.

Other Financial or Institutional Support Systems

The utilization of appropriate resources is often linked directly to the patient's financial status. Prior to determining a referral, assessment of the patient's ability to pay for services is needed. Some agencies require full payment of fees, some have payment plans, while others have sliding fee schedules. Many community agencies only offer their services to people of low income. It is the physician's responsibility to determine, prior to referral, the financial constraints of the patient and the fiscal policy of the agency. The physician will also want to keep in mind such sources of support as Veterans Administration benefits, Health and Welfare agencies, union membership, church organizations, and family resources. The physician may act as a patient advocate with various agencies to insure appropriate support.

Case History

Mr. R was placed in a nursing home under the auspices of the Veterans Administration after the diagnosis of brain tumor was made. Limitation of his coverage was set at 6 months. The physician determined that the needs of the patient and family would extend much longer than the 6-month period of time, but that he could eventually be cared for at home. Acting as a patient advocate with the Veterans Administration, the physician faciliated the establishment of the patient's eligibility for "aide and attendant care." Following his 6-month eligibility period at the nursing home, the patient was transferred home with continued Veterans Administration benefits that allowed for his care.

Other Assessments

To properly assess the needs of the patient, the physician needs to consider the patient's age, degree and type of disability, and community geographic location. These are all contributing factors in locating an appropriate community resource. In most communities there are specific agencies serving target populations, such as senior citizens, adolescents, and preschool children. Many agencies will only serve patients residing in a specific geographic location. Other agencies are dedicated specifically to provide services for limited and identified disabilities (Table 19-1).

FACILITATING THE REFERRAL

It is only after a complete needs assessment by the family physician that the process of referral begins. Facilitation of a referral requires the physician to be aware of the application process employed by the prospective agency. The physician will need to know if a letter of referral is needed, what information about the patient is expected, and how the needs of both the patient and the agency can best be facilitated. In many cases, it is advisable for the physician to encourage the patient or patient's family to make the initial contact with an agency. This allows the patient an independent opportunity to decide whether to proceed with the application process.[3, 4]

Weller et al. have stressed the need for the physician to maintain continuity with the patient and with the resources.[5] The physician can

TABLE 19-1.   Available Community Resources

Health Care—General
Health Departments
Child Health Clinics
Immunization Clinics
Family Planning Clinics
Tuberculosis Clinics
WIC (Women – Infants – Children) food supplement programs
Public Health Nurses
Children's Dental Services
Children and Youth Clinics
Venereal Disease Clinics

Home Care Agencies
Visiting Nurse Service (and other Medicare and state-certified home health agencies)
Medical Personnel Pool
Manpower Medical Services
Homemakers, Inc.
We Sit Better
Others—usually listed in the Yellow Pages under "Nurses"

Medical Equipment and Surgical Supplies
Private companies listed in the phone directory

Social Services—Public Agencies
Health and Welfare Agencies

Division of Public Assistance
Information and Referral Service
Financial Aid
ADC (Aid to Families with Dependent Children)
GAU (General Assistance to the Unemployed)
Food Stamp Program
Medicaid
Case Work Services
Child Care
Homemaker Services
Child Welfare Services (foster care)
Child Protective Services

State Services for the Blind
Bureau of Developmental Disabilities
Employment Services
Job Services
Unemployment Compensation

TABLE 19-1.   Continued.

Counseling Services

Community Mental Health Centers
Individual
Group
Day Treatment
Crisis Outreach Teams
Growth Groups, e.g., Family Life Education

Family Agencies
(should be members of the Family Service Association of America)
Individual
Group
Family Life Education classes

Other
Sexual Assault Centers
Private Practice Counselors, e.g., Psychiatrists, Psychologists, and Social
Workers

Disease-Related Agencies

American Cancer Society
Cancer Life-Line
American Diabetes Association
Cerebral Palsy Center
Childbirth Education Association
Association for Retarded Citizens
Multiple Sclerosis Association
Muscular Dystrophy Association
Spastic Children's Clinic
State Lung Association
Speech and Hearing Clinics

Short-Term Emergency Assistance

American Red Cross (disaster relief; servicemen's families)
Salvation Army Welfare Service
Milk Fund (funds for food in households with children)

Informational and Referral Services

United Way
Department of Social and Health Services
Easter Seals (Handicapped Services)
Senior Services (over 60 age group)
Alcoholism Agency
Center for Addiction Services
Medicare Information—Social Security Office
Crisis Clinics

I hereby give permission for a mutual exchange of information between

_____

_____

Street address   City   State   Zip code
and _____, M.D. including any and all
information regarding the history, diagnostic, and treament records and similar
information from the record of

_____

Patient Name   Patient Birthdate

Approximate dates of service _____

_____

Signature of Person Giving Consent

_____   _____

Relationship   Date

_____   _____

Signature of Witness   Title

(Name of Physician)

FIGURE 19-1.   Consent For Mutual Exchange of Information.

facilitate this process by utilizing a "consent for mutual exchange of information" at the time of the initial contact (Figure 19-1). This will
provide the physician with the opportunity to evaluate the patient's progress and be prepared to make changes based on the needs of the patient.

An inadequate assessment of need by the physician, an inappropriate selection of the agency, an unwillingness of the patient to accept the
prescribed help, bureaucratic realities of long waiting lists, cumbersome
rules and regulations, and difficult eligibility requirements all play a
detrimental role to the successful utilization of community agencies.
Tables 19-2 and 19-3 summarize the steps that can help to avoid these
pitfalls.

EVALUATING COMMUNITY AGENCIES

Kane et al.[6] emphasize that an appropriate evaluation of a community
health agency is based on the agency's stated objectives, goals, and
achievements as measured by how effectively and efficiently it functions.
Although physicians do not have extensive time available to conduct in-

TABLE 19-2.   Facilitating the Use of Community Agencies

1.0   Identify the specific physical and/or psychosocial problem.
2.0   Identify the patient's (and/or family's) perception of the problem.

    2.1   What does the patient or family want to do about it?
    2.2   What has already been done?
    2.3   What resources have been used in the past?

3.0   Identify the patient's available resources.

    3.1   Personal, family, and social support systems
    3.2   Financial resources available

4.0   Determine community resources available.

    4.1   Patient's eligibility, e.g. financial, age, geographic location, disability, etc.
    4.2   Accessibility to the patient
    4.3   Patient's ability to meet a "fee for service" requirement
    4.4   Waiting period
    4.5   Will the services be available to meet the patient's needs?

5.0   Function as a facilitator in the referral process.
6.0   Act as an advocate if needed.
7.0   Determine success of referral

    7.1   Utilize a "consent for mutual exchange of information."
    7.2   Obtain feedback from patient, family, and agency.

---

depth evaluations of community resources, useful evaluation can be accomplished by considering the following questions:

1. Is the resource sanctioned by a qualified national or governmental group? Agencies sanctioned by the federal or state governments as well as United Way must meet specific standards and remain fiscally accountable to their funding sources. Agencies also can be sanctioned by schools of social work as being acceptable for placement of students.

2. Is the resource included in approved information and referral lists? United Way, state and county departments of health and welfare, and crisis centers will often sponsor and maintain information and referral services that provide information regarding acceptable and appropriate agencies. These listings can also clarify the areas of service offered by an agency.

3. What is the experience of other health professionals with the re-

TABLE 19-3.   Pitfalls to Avoid in Making Referrals

1. Making cursory assessments.
2. Lack of patient and/or family involvement in the decision for referral.
3. Lack of preparing patients as to what to expect.
4. Lack of coordination between health and welfare providers.
5. Being unaware of changes in agencies, e.g. policies, procedures, programs, locations, etc.
6. Lack of patient advocacy, where needed.
7. Not meeting agency requirements for referral.
8. Not recognizing that referrals in complex situations are time-consuming.

source? Hospital social workers, visiting nurses, public health nurses, psychologists, nutritionists, and other allied health professionals may be able to provide helpful evaluations to the physician. This underscores the need for the physician to work closely with others in the community.

4. What has the physician's own experience been? The final and possibly the best method of evaluation is the physician's own experience with particular agencies. By appropriately facilitating referrals, maintaining a coordinating role, encouraging ongoing exchanges of information, and judging the outcome of the referral, each physician will select high quality community resources. The only impediment to this is time, and therefore experience, within the community.

RURAL COMMUNITY SERVICES

With a significant number of family physicians establishing their practices in rural communities, attention to the resources commonly found in

**TABLE 19-4.   Services Common to
Rural Communities**

Public Health and Welfare Services*
Alcoholism Programs*
Senior Services (may be sporadic)
Home Care Agency
Crisis Line
Information and Referral (may be part
    of Crisis Line or United Way)
Volunteer groups

* May have representatives in the area part-time

such communities is appropriate. The range of agencies which appear in Table 19-1 of this chapter is generally representative of those found in urban centers. In recent years, rural health and public programs, in cooperation with county health and welfare agencies, have begun to develop resources for rural communities. Common examples of such resources are listed in Table 19-4. Usually these resources are provided as branch offices of urban agencies, and they are staffed on a part-time basis during the week. Expansion of these services can be aided by the practicing physician who encourages nearby agencies to establish branch offices. The physician can also be instrumental in organizing volunteer services that provide transportation, clothing, emergency housing, and crisis intervention.

REFERENCES

1. Schubert M: *Interviewing in Social Work Practice: An Introduction.* New York: Council on Social Work Education, 1971
2. Weller MD, Ruth DH, Seller RM: Effective use of patient resources: A training service for family physicians. J Fam Pract 4:515–20, 1977
3. Brammer LM: *The Helping Relationship: Process and Skills.* Englewood Cliffs, New Jersey: Prentice-Hall, 1973
4. Lamb L: The social worker as a teacher of family practice residents. Can Fam Phys 21:117, 1975
5. Weller: op. cit., pp. 515–16
6. Kane RL, Henson R, Deniston OL: "Program Evaluation: Is It Worth It?" In Kane RL, ed: *The Challenge of Community Medicine.* New York: Springer Publishing, 1974

INDEX

INDEX

A-B-C model of behavior, 173–174, 178

Abandonment, as a crisis, 21, 22, 25, 73, 78. *See also* Loss

Abramson, E., 266

Academic social sciences, 11–12

Accidents, relating to aging, 58

Accreditation, 7

Acne, 42

Acting out, 98

Active listening, 118

Activity Diary, 180, 182

Acute organic brain syndrome, 166, 167

Adaptability, as basic need of child, 47

Addictions, 12, 269. *See also* specific addiction

Addition, as a crisis, 21, 22, 73, 78

Administrative science, 9

Adolescence
development during, 42–44, 86, 98
and emotional instability, 161
and psychotherapy, 240–241
reactions to illness during, 45–46
and sexual identity, 233

Adrenalin, as cause of anxiety, 161

Adult development, 49–66, 69, 98
changes during, 59–64
and role of the physician, 64–66
stages of, 52–59, 64–66, 69, 241–244, 267

Advice, direct, 236

Affective state
change in, and crisis state, 222
and evaluation of mental status, 160–162

Aging, 58, 160, 267

Agism, 57

Agitated depression, 165

Alcohol
  and euphoria, 162
  and evaluation of mental status, 159
Alcoholism
  and female hysterical personality disorder, 138
  and group assertion techniques, 266, 269
  in mid-life crisis, 55
Alliances, in family therapy, 257
Alzheimer's disease, 160
American Academy of Family Physicians, 5. See also American Academy of General Practice
Commission on Education, 6
American Academy of General Practice, 4. See also American Academy of Family Physicians
Committee on Requirements for Certification (CORC), 6
Mental Health Committee, 5–6
American Board of Family Practice, 6
American Medical Association, 4
American Orthopsychiatric Association, 247–248
American Psychiatric Association, 5
Amphetamines, as cause of anxiety, 161
Analytic oriented therapy, 205
Analytic-psychologic psychiatrists, 204
Anger, 125, 134
Animal psychology, 11, 207
Anthropology, 11, 99
Antianxiety drugs, 208
Antidepressants, tricyclic, 138
Anxiety, 208
  causes of, 161, 208
  and crisis, 221
  definition of, 161
  and depression, 127
  guilt grief reaction, 133
  limits of, 238
  medication for, 208
  somatic symptoms of, 165, 208
Anxiety reaction, acute, 125–127

Apathy, 161–162
Arthritis, 56, 58
Associations, loose, 159, 163
Asthma, 269
Autism, childhood, 12
Autistic thinking, 163
Autonomic symptoms, 207
Autonomy versus doubt and shame, stage of, 84

Balint, Michael, 8, 15, 100, 101, 211, 212, 231, 236
Balint's seminars, 8, 15, 102
Bart, Pauline, 212
Beck Depression Inventory, 190, 194
Behavior modification, 12, 100
Behavioral science
  education in, 4, 265
  historical roots of, in family practice, 4–9
  intellectual roots of, 9–13
  model of, 15–26
Beitman, B., 234
Benign/competent therapist model, 232
Benjamin, A., 120
Benzodiazepines, 138
Bettelheim, Bruno, 12
Bill, A., 229
Biofeedback, 12
Biomedical model, 16, 99
Bipolar affective disease, 95, 157
Birley, J., 220
Bishop, F. M., 120
Blake, A., 266
Block, D. A., 250
Bloom, B., 219
Body language, 113–114, 118, 165, 211
Bowen, M., 250
British general practice, 7–8
Brown, G., 220
Bureaucratic institutions, 100
Burnell, G. M., 267
Byrne, P. S., 109, 121

Cadoret, R. J., 234
Caffeine, as cause of anxiety, 161
Cancer
  in advanced adulthood, 58
  and depression, 168
  family health groups for, 266
  and personality change, 157
Caplan, G., 217, 219, 220
Cardiovascular disease
  in advanced adulthood, 58
  family health groups for, 269
  in mid-life crisis, 55
  in middle adulthood, 56
  and personality type, 197
Carmichael, L., 7, 79
Catatonia, 96
Catharsis, emotional, 233–234
Central nervous system diseases
  and anxiety, 161
  and apathy, 161–162
  and delirium, 162
  and depression, 168
  and emotional instability, 161
  and euphoria, 162
Certification, for general practitioners,
  6
Change, and crisis, 220
Chaplain, hospital, 8
Chess, S., 32
Child abuse and neglect, 33
Child development, 31–47, 83, 84–86,
  98, 266. See also Children
Childbirth, 267, 269
Children. See also Child development
  basic needs of, 46–47
  cognitive development of, 34
  and death and dying, 46
  and discipline, 41–42
  and emotional instability, 161
  measuring behavior of, 35–36, 37–
  40
  and play, 36, 41
  reactions of, to illness, 45, 46
  social behavior of, 41
  treatment of, in family health
  groups, 266

Chronic diseases
  family health groups for, 269
  in middle adulthood, 56
  in preparation for retirement stage,
  57
  problems of, 100
  transference-countertransference,
  101
Chronic organic brain syndrome, 166–
  167
Chronic pain, self-monitoring of, 175,
  176–177, 180, 182
Chronological age, 60
Cincinnati, University of, School of
  Medicine, 8
Clinical pastoral education, 8
Clinical psychology, 11
Closed questions, 115
Coalitionary process, in family ther-
  apy, 257
Cognition. See Intellectual functioning
Cognitive development, 34
Commonwealth Fund, 249
Communication. See Doctor–patient
  relationship,   communication
  in; Family, communication in;
  Nonverbal communication
Communications theory, in family
  therapy, 12
Community mental health centers, 6.
  See also Community resources
Community resources, 279–288
Compliance, 99. See also Noncompli-
  ance
Compound questions, 115
Compulsive behavior, 159
Condition, differentiating from prob-
  lem, 118–119
Confabulation, 160, 163
Conscience, 41
Consent for mutual exchange of infor-
  mation, 285
Continuous case seminars, 8, 15, 102
Contraception, 43
Conversion syndromes, 164
Cooperative play, 41

Coping, 22, 218, 219, 220, 221, 222, 226, 227
  and adult development, 62–63, 65–66
  assessment of, 97–98
  maladaptive, 100
Cornell University Medical College, 249
Coronary prone personality, 197
Counseling, 124, 138, 204
Countertransference, 10, 15, 101–102, 113, 156, 213. *See also* Transference
Creativity, 61
Crisis, 20–23
  case illustrations of, 222–226
  definitions of, 20, 68, 217–219, 220
  and family, 68, 73, 77, 78, 79, 99–100, 141–143, 145, 148–149, 224, 227, 228
  identity, 43, 53–54
  mid-life, 54–56
  nonnormative, 20, 21, 22, 73
  normative, 20, 21, 22, 73, 240
  relationship of, to stressful life events, 219–221
  stages of, 221–222
Crisis intervention, 217–229, 269
Crying, 169
Crystalized intelligence, 61
Cultural factors, 210. *See also* Ethnicity; Social class; Social factors
Cultural norms, 96

Death and dying. *See also* Grief
  and children, 46
  and crisis intervention, 225–226
  and interviewing, 132–134
  literature on, 8
  and maturity, 243
  as nonnormative crisis, 73
Defense mechanisms, 98, 112, 205. *See also specific name*
Déjà vu, 164
Delirium, 161, 162

Delusions, 95
Dementia, 158, 160, 161, 162
Demoralization, as a crisis, 21, 22, 25, 73, 78
Denial, 98, 112
Denver Developmental Screening Test, 190, 194–195
Depression
  and abandonment, 145
  agitated, 162
  and crisis, 221
  and diabetes, 96
  diagnosis of, 167–168
  and family development, 79
  and fear, 161
  and interviewing, 127–129
  and mental status examination, 161, 167–169
  in mid-life crisis, 55
  and pancreatic carcinoma, 157
  and personal appearance, 159
  and preparation for retirement, 57
  postpartum, 79
  post retirement, 79
Deutsch, C. B., 267
Development examination, 35–36, 37–40
Developmental framework, clinical applications of, 83–92
Developmental psychology, 12
Developmental quotient, 35–36
Developmental stages. *See also* Adult development; Child development
  concept of, 7, 10, 12
  and psychotherapy, 240–244
Developmental stresses, 220, 223–224
Diabetes, 56, 58, 96, 98, 269
Diagnosis
  in family medicine, 265
  in psychotherapy, 237–240
Diarrhea, 164
Diet monitoring form, 174
Direct questioning, and meaning of illness to patient, 99
Directive-organic psychiatrists, 204

Disease
new, and psychological problems, 209
and weakening of coping skills, 219
Disease problems versus illness problems, 96–97
Displacement, 98
Dissociation, 98, 169
Divorce, 54, 73. *See also* Marriage, crisis in
Doctor, His Patient and the Illness, The, 8
Doctor–patient contact categories, 237–239
Doctor–patient relationship. *See also* Physician
and biomedical model, 16
communication in, 57, 60, 98, 99, 113–114, 118–119, 124, 125, 168, 211–212, 236
and female hysterical personality disorder, 135–137
and medical behavioral science, 15–16
in mid-life crisis, 55
and personal life of physician, 136
and psychoanalysis, 10
and psychotherapy, 206, 215, 232, 233
quality of, 111, 114, 124
symbolic nature of, 10. *See also* Countertransference; Transference
teaching about, 8
and therapeutic negotiation, 98–99
and touch, 114, 168, 206–207
Doctors Talking To Patients, 109
Dreams, 85
Dress, and evaluation of mental status, 159
Drug(s). *See also specific name*
abuse of
iatrogenic, 137–138
in mid-life crisis, 55
as cause of anxiety, 161
and evaluation of mental status, 159

Drug(s) (*cont.*)
withdrawal of, and delirium, 162
Drug history, 157
Duration measures, 180, 181, 182
Duvall, E. M., 71, 72, 73
Dyads, 11

Education
clinical pastoral, 8
medical
in behavioral science, 4, 265
continuing, 6, 227
in educational psychology, 7
in psychiatry, 6
in psychotherapy, 8, 206
special, 8
Educational groups. *See* Family Health Groups
Educational psychology, 7, 12
Eisenberg, K., 98
Emesis, 164
Emotional catharsis, 233–234
Emotional instability, and central nervous system lesions, 161
Empty-nest syndrome, 56, 222
Enelow, A. J., 120
Engineering, 11
Engle, G. L., 96
Enmeshment, 150
Environment, and child development, 31–34
Ephedrine, as cause of anxiety, 161
Epilepsy, 96
Erikson, Erik, 12, 56, 83, 85, 86, 87, 92, 242, 243
Ethnicity. *See also* Cultural factors; Social class; Social factors
and illness beliefs, 98, 99
and treatment objectives, 98, 99, 101
Ethnology, 11, 207
Euphoria, and evaluation of mental status, 162
Excitement, and evaluation of mental status, 162
Eye contact, in medical interview, 114

Facial expressions
  and evaluation of mental status,
    161, 165
  in medical interview, 114
  of physician, 211
Families In Crisis, 68
Family
  communication in, 19, 20, 23
  conflicts, 55
  and crisis, 73, 76, 77, 78, 79, 99–
    100, 141–142, 145, 148–149,
    224, 227, 228
  definitions of, 69–70, 142, 143, 144,
    145
  development, 24, 25, 67–81, 98
  dysfunctional, 19, 20, 141, 142, 144
  function
    assessment of, 141–151
    data base, 23–25
    definition of, 142, 143–144
    and stress of sickness, 99–100
  functional, 19, 141–142
  homeostasis, 249, 255
  interactional responses in, 142, 143,
    146, 224
  involvement of, in patient care, 148
  life cycle. *See* Family, development
  nuclear, 69, 146
  resources of, 19, 20, 22, 23, 24,
    100, 142, 148, 226–227
  structure of, 42, 69, 145, 146
Family APGAR, 23, 24, 144, 146–150
Family charting system, 261
Family counseling, 129–132
Family Function Index, 146, 147, 148
Family Health Groups, 265–276
Family history, 127, 128, 261
Family Medicine, 95
*Family Medicine: Principles and Ap-
  plications*, 266
Family therapy, 11, 235, 247–262
Family tree, 143
Fear(s). *See also* Phobias
  definition of, 161
  of dying, 46
  and evaluation of mental status,
    161, 163

Fear(s) (*cont.*)
  of strangers, 33
  underlying complaint, 124, 125
Fees
  for Family Health Groups, 271, 272
  for psychotherapy, 205–206
Feighner, J. P., 209
Feinstein, A., 210
Feldman, H., 25, 68
Female hysterical personality disorder,
    134–138
Fetus, environmental influences on, 32
Fisch, R., 257
Fluid intelligence, 61
Focused questions, 115
Fordyce, W. E., 180
Foundations of Psychopathology, 134
Frank, Jerome, 233
Frankl, Victor, 13
Free-floating anxiety, 221
Freedom, as basic need of child, 47
Freud, S., 204, 205, 266, 234
Fried, Barbara, 55
Friedman, W. H., 267, 269
Friendships, 63
Frequency counts, 175–179
Frigidity, 164
Froelich, R. E., 120
Fromm, Erich, 13
Functional age, 60
Functional analysis of behavior, 173–
    174, 178
Functional status, 221, 222

Game theory, 11, 12
Gastrointestinal symptoms, biofeed-
    back for, 12
Gauron, E. F., 271, 272
General intelligence, 61
General practice
  British, 7–8
  traditional, 4–5
Generativity versus stagnation, stage
  of, 86, 242
Genetic relationships, 143
Gestalt psychology, 13

Glasser, L. N., 68
Glasser, P. H., 68
Good, B., 98
Gordon, Thomas, 118
Gould, R. L., 69
Grace, N. T., 261
Graph paper, for use in self-monitoring, 177
Greer, S., 229
Grief. *See also* Death and dying
  interviewing patient with, 132–134
  pathologic, 134
Group process, 11, 274–275
Group therapy, 11. *See also specific name*
Groups, Family Health. *See* Family Health Groups
Growth, in adolescence, 42
Guerin, P. J., 250
Guilt
  and depression, 129
  in grief reaction, 133, 134

Habits, behavior modification for, 12
Hallucinations, 95, 158, 164
Havens, Leston, 203
Havighurst, Robert, 12
Head injury, 161, 162
Headache, 164
  biofeedback for, 12
  and psychological problems, 207
  self-monitoring of, 180, 183
Healing process, belief in, 233
Health
  in advanced adulthood, 58
  in early adulthood, 54
  and life style, 62–63
  in mid-life crisis, 55
  in middle adulthood, 56
  and personality, 62–63
  and stage of leaving home for real, 54
Health beliefs, 16
Health maintenance, 101
Hearing, 60
Heart attacks. *See* Cardiovascular dis-

Heart attacks (*cont.*)
    ease; Coronary prone personality
Henderson, L. J., 11
Hertzler, A. E., 5
Hierarchy of personal needs, 13
Hill, R., 20
History
  and crisis intervention, 228
  family, 127, 128, 261
  and mental status examination, 156, 157
  in psychotherapy, 214, 235
  second-party, 158, 160
  sexual, 119–120, 214
Hollingshead, A. B., 204
Holmes-Rahe Life Stress Scale, 197
Holmes, T. H., 73, 197, 220
Homeostasis, 217–218
  family, 249, 255
Homicidal thoughts, 163
Hommans, George, 11
Horse and Buggy Doctor, 5
Horwitz, L., 269
Hospital, interviewing patient in, 110
Hospitalization, of children, 33, 45
Hostility, in grief reaction, 133, 134
Humanistic psychology, 12–13
Huygen, F. J., 20
Hypertension, 12, 269
Hyperthyroidism, 208
Hyperventilation syndrome, 125–127
Hypnagogic experience, 164
Hypnopompic experience, 164
Hysteria, 95, 96, 169–170
Hysterical blindness, 164
Hysterical paralysis, 164, 169–170
Hysterical personality disorder, female, 134–138

Iatrogenic drug abuse, 137–138
Iatrogenic stress, 102
Iatrotrophic stimulus, 210, 211
Identified patient, 253–254
Identity
  occupational, 44, 86
  sexual, 233

Identity crisis, 43, 53–54
Illness
    adolescent reaction to, 45–46
    children's reaction to, 45, 46
    meaning of, to patient, 99
    serious, as nonnormative crisis, 23
Illness behavior, 16
Illness beliefs, 98–99
Illness metaphors, 212
Illness problems, 96–97
    assessment of, 97–102
    versus disease problems, 96–97
Imaginary people, 36
Imitative play, 36, 41
Immediate recall memory, 159
Impotence, 164
Industry versus inferiority, stage of, 85–86
Infancy, 84. *See also* Child development
Influenza, as cause of depression, 168
Initiative versus guilt, stage of, 85
Insight, 165
Integrity versus despair, stage of, 57, 87, 243
Intellectual functioning
    and adult development, 61–62
    in evaluation of mental status, 162–163, 164, 165
    loss of, 158
    tests of, 162–164, 194, 196, 197. *See also specific test*
    and social class, 34
International Journal of Group Psychotherapy, 276
Interview (ing)
    and the difficult patient, 123–138
    engagement, 234
    initial screening, for Family Health Groups, 270–271
    and psychological problems, 210, 214–215
    skills, 109–121, 123–124
Intimacy and isolation, stage of, 86
Involutional melancholia, 168
Irritable colon, 164

Jackson, Don, 249
Jamais vu, 164
Jelly, E., 267
Jelly, P., 267
Jenkins, C. D., 197
Judgment, and evaluation of mental status, 164

Kane, R. L., 285
Kaufman, E., 229
Kierkegaard, Soren, 13
Kleinman, A., 98
Kluckholn, F. R., 22
Korsakow's psychosis, 160
Kramer, N., 267
Kuypers, J. A., 62

Lamaze method of childbirth, 267
Langsley, D., 227, 239
LaPerriere, K., 250
Leading questions, 115
Learning disorders, 12, 266
Learning theory, 7
Levine, M., 204
Lieberman, M. A., 270, 273
Lindemann, Eric, 132
Linguistics, 11
Lipowski, Z. J., 99
Listening–responding skills, 116–118, 121
Long, B., 109
Long-term memory, 62
Loss, and depression, 128–129, 168. *See also* Abandonment
Luisada, P. V., 135
Lung diseases, 58
Lupus erythematosus, 157

Maas, H. S., 62
Macy Study, The, 249
Maladaptive behavior, 221
Mania, 161, 162
Manic-depression, 95, 157
Manual dexterity, 60

Marriage(s)
  crisis in, 129–132. *See also* Divorce
  in early adulthood, 54
  and maturation, 130–132
  in middle adulthood, 56
  as normative crisis, 73
  satisfaction with, 68
Marriage counseling, 11
Maslow, Abraham, 13
Maternal–infant bonding, 32–33
Mathematics, 11
Mauksch, H. O., 16
May, Rollo, 13
McWhinney, I. R., 237, 238
Mead, George Herbert, 11
Medalie, J., 261
Medical anthropology, 99
Medical care
  fragmentation of, 5
  impersonality of, 5
Medical psychology, 9–10, 11, 12, 14
Medical social work, 11
Memory function, 61–62
Memory testing, 159–160, 162, 165
Men
  climacteric in, 61
  death rate of, 55, 56
  early American view of stages in
    lives of, 49, 51, 52
  and hysterical personality disorder,
    135
  suicide of, 57
Menarche, 42
Menopause, 61, 269
Mental health, 6, 11
Mental illness, 221, 226, 231. *See also*
  specific disorder
Mental retardation, 12
Mental status examination, 128, 155–
  170
Metabolic diseases, and delirium, 162
Metabolic encephalopathy, 96
Metaphors, illness, 212
Michigan State University, 7
Middle-Age Crisis, The, 55
Miles, M. B., 270
Miller, F. G. W., 20

Millis Commission, 4
Mini-Mental State (MMS), 164
Minnesota Multiphasic Personality In-
  ventory (MMPI), 190, 191,
  192, 195
Minuchin, S., 150
Mood, and evaluation of mental status,
  161–162, 165
Mortality rates, 55, 56, 58
Motor behavior, and evaluation of
  mental status, 159
Multiple sclerosis, 161, 162
Murdock, G. P., 142
Myers, J., 220

National Conference on Family Life,
  71, 72
National Institute of Mental Health
  (NIMH), 6
Natural disasters, and crisis interven-
  tion, 226
Nemiah, John, 134
Neologisms, 163
Neugarten, B. L., 63
New York Hospital, 249
Nicotine, as cause of anxiety, 161
Noncompliance, 98, 119. *See also*
  Compliance
Nonnormative crisis, 20, 21, 22, 73
Nonverbal communication, 113–114,
  118, 121, 136, 165, 211
Normative crisis, 20, 21, 22, 73, 240
Nurture, and the family, 143

Obesity, 12, 56
Observation. *See also* Self-monitoring
  and meaning of illness, 99
  in medical interview, 113
  in mental status examination, 165
Obsessions, 159, 163
Omnibus testing, 61
Open-ended questions, 114–115, 123–
  124
Organic brain syndrome, 95, 166–167
Organizational activities, and histori-

Organizational activities (*cont.*)
cal roots of behavioral science, 5–7
"Organizing the illness," 211
Orientation, and evaluation of mental status, 159, 160, 165
Osler, W., 109

Pain, chronic. *See* Chronic pain, self-monitoring of
Pancreas, carcinoma of, 157
Parad, H., 219, 227
Paranoid thinking, 58–59
Parent–adolescent relationship, 44
Parenting techniques, 267
Parents, single, 42
Pareto, W., 11
Passive-hostile behavior, 98
Past memory, 159
Pastoral education, clinical, 8
Pathologic grief reaction, 134
Patient(s). *See also* Compliance; Doctor–patient relationship; Noncompliance
assessment of problem by, and referral to community agency, 280–282
behavior of, 237–240
characteristics of, and problems for physician, 212–213
dependent, 138
dissatisfaction of, 98
financial status of, 281–282
manipulative, 136, 137
metaphors of, 212
new, and use of Family APGAR, 148
satisfaction, 121
Patient education, 121, 124, 126, 204, 222, 233
Patients Have Families, 249
Paykel, E., 220
Peak experiences, 13
Peckham Experience, The, 248–249
Peele, Roger, 135
Peer group, adolescent, 43

Perception, disorders of, 164
Perls, Fritz, 13
Perseveration, 163
Person, psychology of, 12–13
Personality, 112
and health, 62–63
influences on, 31
and life style, 62–63
Personality change, and metastatic carcinoma, 157
Personality disorders, 33, 96. *See also specific disorder*
Pheochromocytoma, 208
Phobias, 95. *See also* Fear(s)
Physical capabilities, 57, 59–60
Physical changes, in adolescence, 59–60
Physical examination, 209, 214
Physically handicapped, 260
Physician. *See also* Doctor–patient relationship; Education, medical
advanced adults visits to, 58, 64–66
apostolic function of, 212
appearance of, 114
and family development, 78–79, 81
feelings of, 156. *See also* Countertransference
mental health of, 6
personal life of, 136
personality of, 100, 244
prejudices of, 113
reaction of, to secret information, 211
as referee, 130
as role model, 233
sexual knowledge of, 130
specializations of, 5
Piaget, Jean, 12, 34
Pioneer Health Center, 248
Pless, B., 146, 147, 148
Pomerleau, O., 266
"Pop" psychology, 102
Postencephalitic Parkinsonism, 162
Postpartum depression, 79
Post retirement depression, 79
Posture, 114
Pratt, J. H., 266

Pratt, L., 143
Pregnancy, 32, 73
Presenile dementia, 160
Problem, differentiating from condition, 118–119
Problem-solving, 62, 221
Projection, 98
Projective tests, 192, 194, 196. *See also specific test*
Psychiatric interview, 117
Psychiatrist, 129, 204, 206, 231–232. *See also* Referrals, to mental health professionals
Psychiatry, in medical education, 6
Psychoactive drugs, 228
Psychoanalysis, 9–10, 12, 205, 266
Psychological problems
    of advanced adulthood, 58–59
    identification of, 207–210
Psychological testing, 189–198
Psychomotor restlessness, in agitated depression, 162
Psychopaths, 162
Psychosis, 95, 157, 226
Psychosocial crisis, 20–25, 141–142
Psychosocial problems
    assessment of, 95–106
    common, 124–125, 138
    in mid-life crisis, 55
    and model of behavioral science, 17–19
Psychotherapy
    compensation for, 205–206
    curative factors in, 232–234
    definition of, 204–205, 231
    education in, 8, 206
    in family practice setting, 100, 205–207, 210–215
Psychotropic drugs, 235
Puberty, 42. *See also* Adolescence

Questioning, in medical interview, 114–115

Rage, 162

Rahe, R., 220
Rakel, R., 121
Ransom, D. C., 69
Rapoport, L., 217
Rawlings, E. I., 217, 272
Reaction formation, 98, 112
Reactive sadness, 167
Reality testing, 95
Reassurance, 124, 222, 233
Recent memory, 159
Redlich, F. C., 204
Referrals
    to community agencies, 279–288
    to mental health professionals, 100, 130, 213, 215, 237, 244, 262, 269
Reframing, in family therapy, 257
Regier, D. A., 231
Regression, 85
Religion, 12–13, 43
Repression, 112
Resources. *See* Community resources; Family, resources of; Support systems
Retirement, 73, 79, 222
Richardson, Henry B., 142, 249
Rogers, C. R., 232
Rogers, Carl, 13
Role
    sex, 33
    sick, 99, 100–101
Role change, 24. *See also* Status change
Role diffusion, 86
Role model, physician as, 233
Role theory, 11
Rollins, B. C., 25, 68
Rorschach Inkblots, 190
Rotter Incomplete Sentence Blank, 190, 194, 196, 197
Rubin, Stella, 135
Rural community agencies, 287–288

Sadness, 167
Satterwhite, B., 146, 147, 148
Schizophrenia, 95

Schizophrenia (*cont.*)
  catatonic, 162
  and dress, 159
  and loose associations, 159
  and temporal lobe epilepsy, 96
School, as socializing agent, 85–86
Screening inventory, 35–36, 37–40
Security, as basic need of child, 47
Self
  infant's awareness of, 33
  as object of study, 11, 12
Self actualization, 13
Self-care, 98, 101
Self-criticism, 41
Self-monitoring, 171–187
Self-rating depression scale, 169
Semantics, 11
Senile dementia, 160
Sensory organs, ailments of, 58, 60
Sensory perceptions, 60
Separation, as nonnormative crisis, 73
Separation anxiety, 33, 85, 133
Sex roles, 33
Sexual activity, 43–44, 60–61
Sexual deviance, 95
Sexual history, 119–120, 214
Sexual identity, 233
Sexual interest, 164
Sexual knowledge, 43–44, 233
  of physician, 130
Sheehy, Gail, 55
Shipley-Hartford Retreat Scale. *See* Shipley Institute of Living Scale
Shipley Institute of Living Scale, 194, 197
Short-term memory, 62
Sibling rivalry, 33, 85
Sick role, 99, 100–101
Single parents, 42
Skinner, B. F., 12
Slavson, S. R., 268, 269
Sleep disturbances, 164–165, 168
Sluzki, C., 251
Small Group Behavior, 276
Small groups, 11, 274–275. *See also* Family Health Groups

Smell, sense of, 60
Smilkstein, G., 69
Smith, L. L., 217
Smith, Zilpha D., 247
Social attachments, 63–64
Social class. *See also* Cultural factors; Ethnicity; Social factors
  and illness beliefs, 98
  and intellectual performance, 34, 35
  and treatment objectives, 98, 100
Social factors. *See also* Cultural factors; Ethnicity; Social class
  and physician consultation, 210
  and psychosocial crisis, 25
  taxonomy of, 237, 238, 239–240
Social organizations, 63
Social play, 36
Social problems. *See also* Psychosocial problems
  of advanced adulthood, 59
Social psychology, 11
Social Readjustment Rating Scale, 73, 77
Social sciences, academic, 11–12
Social structure, 96
Society of Teachers of Family Medicine, 7
Sociology, 11
Somatic complaints, 132, 207–208
Somatization, 95, 98, 100, 155, 164–165
Special education, 12
Speech, 159, 266
Spiegel, J. P., 144
Status change, 21, 22, 73, 78. *See also* Role change
Straker, M., 229
Stress
  accidental, 220
  coping with, 218, 219, 220
  and special treatments, 102
Stressful life events. *See also* Crisis
  and the behavioral science model, 19–20
  related to crisis, 219–221
Strokes, 161

"Study of the Family in Sickness and Health Care, The," 249
Success, as basic need of child, 47
Suggestion, role of, 236
Suicidal status, 95
Suicidal thoughts, 163
Support systems, 63, 281. *See also* Family, resources of
Surgery, 223
Sussman, M. B., 143
Swisher, S. N., 120
Symbolic play, 41
Systemic diseases, and mental status, 157
Systems theory, 11, 12

Taste, sense of, 60
Taxonomy of patient behavior, 237–240
Taxonomy of social factors, 237, 238, 239–240
Temperament, 32
Tension-related problems, self-monitoring of, 180–181, 184, 185
Terminally ill, 266
Thematic Apperception Test (TAT), 190
Theory and Practice of Group Psychotherapy, The, 276
Therapeutic negotiations, 98–99
Third force psychology, 13
Thomas, A., 32
Thought content, 163–164
Thought processes, 163
Thyroxine, as cause of anxiety, 161
Touch
    and depressed patient, 168
    in doctor–patient relationship, 114, 168, 206–207
    and psychotherapy, 206–207
    sense of, 60
Tournier, Paul, 13
Towle, Charlotte, 248
Tranquilizers, 55, 138, 208
Transactional analysis, 12
Transference, 10, 15, 101, 112–113,

Transference (*cont.*)
    213, 232, 235–236. *See also* Countertransference
Treatment
    objectives of, 98–99, 101
    special, stress caused by, 102
    and weakening of coping skills, 219
Tricyclic antidepressants, 138
Troll, L. E., 59, 61, 62, 63
Truax, C. B., 232
Trust versus basic mistrust, stage of, 84
Type A personality, 197

Ulcers, 269

Value orientation, 22
Vanderpool, John P., 52, 53, 55, 57
Vandervoort, H. E., 69
Vascular headache, biofeedback for, 12
Vascular surgery, 266
Venereal disease, 43
"Verbatim" method, 8
Vision, 60
Vocabulary of distress, 212
Vocal play, 36

Watzlawick, P., 257
Weakland, J., 257
Wechsler Adult Intelligence Scale (WAIS), 163, 190, 194, 196, 197
Wechsler Intelligence Scale for Children (WISC), 190, 194, 196, 197
Weight problems, 12, 56, 269
Weitzel, W. D., 158
Well-person examinations, 209
Weller, W. D., 282
Willard Committee, 4
Willard Report, 4
Wollersham, J., 266

Women
early American view of stages in
lives of, 49, 50, 52
and female hysterical personality
disorder, 134–138
and mid-life crisis, 55
in middle adulthood, 56
Worby, C. M., 70, 71, 72

Working through, 235

Yalom, I. D., 270, 276

Zung Self-Rating Depression Scale,
190, 193, 194, 195
Zung, W. W., 169